LOVE, LAUGHTER, & MAYHEM

Cindy Keith, RN, BS, CDP

"A Wealth of Wisdom! How I wish I'd had Cindy's practical and crucial advice during the most horrific year of my life as the sole caregiver to my challenging elderly father and sweet but ailing mother, both with early Alzheimer's which went undiagnosed by professionals for over a year!"

--Jacqueline Marcell, author of *Elder Rage* and host of the *Coping with Caregiving* radio show

BookLocker.com, Inc.
2010

Cindy Keith, RN, BS, CDP
E-mail: keithc@mindinmemorycare.com
Website: www.mindinmemorycare.com
151 Fairlawn Avenue
State College, PA 16801

Cover Design by Todd Engel, Engel Creative

Edited by Joyce M. Gilmour

DISCLAIMER

This book is written to provide information to people who care for and care about people who have dementia. It is not meant to be the final word or promise in any given situation since every person and every situation is unique, and will require different interventions--no end result is guaranteed. These stories and the lessons they contain can help guide caregivers, if they choose.

The information in this book is not meant to replace regular contact with a physician to coordinate care, and prescribe medication, if appropriate, for the person with dementia.

Every effort has been made to recount the basic facts for every story and situation, however major changes such as names, gender, and other identifying characteristics have been intentionally made to protect the identity of the families and their loved ones with dementia.

The author and publisher shall have neither liability nor responsibility to any person or entity with respect to any loss or damage caused or alleged to be caused directly or indirectly by the information contained in this book.

DEDICATION

Love, Laughter, & Mayhem is dedicated to my father and all of the other countless people with dementia whom I have known, loved and worked with. Their lives and broken memories have enriched my life and have helped give birth to this book. You are truly a part of me and I am grateful.

ACKNOWLEDGEMENTS

I am blessed to have a number of caring and supportive friends who have listened to my slow, laborious progress with this book. I appreciate your love, prayers, and willingness to lend a sympathetic ear, or advice when I needed it. You know who you are and I thank you from the bottom of my heart. You have helped me become who I am today and I would not want to live this life without you.

To my husband Doug, and Miss Frizz, gratitude for their patience, love, support and not complaining at all those early alarm clocks going off month after month.

To the families and caregivers of all those wonderful elders with dementia in the stories of my book. Thank you for trusting me to help you and for teaching me along the way as we made those journeys together.

To Betsey Eggler for sharing her wonderful dream that became the cover of this book. Sorry for the interrupted sleep Betsey, but I'm eternally grateful for this dream.

To John Bellanti, D.Ed. PCC for his coaching, encouragement and patience that first led me to believe I could actually write a book:
coachingthruthecrossroads.com

To Sylvia Hopkins for her invaluable advice and support.

To Victoria Alexander for the initial editing, and Joyce M. Gilmour for the subsequent multiple edits.

To Angela at BookLocker.com for her cheerful willingness to help and prompt responses to my many questions.

To Todd Engel for suffering through the many ideas and changes I had for the book cover. Thanks for hanging in there with me Todd.

To Sandi and Keith Cunningham for providing the final push to get this book published. Your teachings will last a lifetime and I appreciate it.

To my Mastermind sisters for seeing this publication and the success of this book for me. We'll meet in person some day, but our hearts are already old friends.

To Oprah Winfrey for inspiring me, and so many others, to dream a bigger dream.

TABLE OF CONTENTS

Reflections From The Author

Writing this book has been both a labor of love and a wrenching of my heart. I wanted and needed to tell you the stories about people with dementia that I have known and loved throughout my nursing career. As with every topic in every book, there are many lessons to be learned from the reading of another person's experiences. It is my fervent hope that you will see and learn the lessons contained herein to assist you as you live with and care for an elder with dementia.

I have chosen the subject of dementia for my career because I discovered I'm very good at it, and because it touches my heart in a way nothing else ever has. Nursing is a very broad palate from which to choose a specialty, and my story about Belle in "I Might Have To Kick You Out!" helps you see why I chose to build my business helping people with dementia and their families. I named my business "MIND In Memory Care" (Moving In Nurturing Directions In Memory Care) because nurturing is what I'm all about, and it's what I believe every person who lives with or works with a person with dementia must be all about in order to safely and effectively interact with these wonderful elders. I believe nurturing can be taught to those willing to learn, and I spend a great deal of time educating people who work in the facilities that house our loved ones with dementia. What better way to illustrate the best or worst way to handle a touchy interaction with an elder with dementia than to tell you a story about what I have experienced? Sometimes there are no answers and sometimes you will choose the wrong way, but you will always learn from it, and hopefully that learning will make you a better caregiver or partner to that loved one with dementia. The struggle is as necessary as the mistakes are inevitable, and what I want you to take away from reading this book is the knowledge that you're not alone in those struggles or those mistakes. There really can be good times ahead with your loved one, and you will learn to recognize and build upon them as they occur.

I feel it is very important for you to allow humor into your life as you live and work in the world of dementia. You can learn how to create many wonderful moments with your loved one, and when that person dies, you will have countless memories to warm your battered heart and bring a smile to your sad face. You can learn to live in the moment in your loved one's mind and see the world through their eyes so that you can make their world a nicer place, and in doing so, also make your own world a calmer and better place. These are the things I want my stories and the lessons they contain to do for you.

Cindy Keith, RN, BS, CDP
State College, PA

The Diagnosis

"I'm sorry I have to tell you this, Cindy, but based on your tests, I believe you have Alzheimer's disease."

I wonder how I would react if I heard those words? What emotions would I experience, and what would I say? How would *you* react if you were the patient sitting in front of that doctor?

Because I like to think I'm an intelligent, logical, and relatively calm person who reacts in a controlled and sensible way during a crisis, I like to believe I would meet that slow death sentence with unflinching courage. After all, I am a nurse who has had lots of experience with crisis situations, and it just doesn't look good when nurses go to pieces in times of crisis. Then again, I might just scream profanities and stomp out of the office never to return to be cared for by such an idiot person. I just don't know; nobody knows what their reaction would be to such devastating news until it actually comes about. But there's also another reason I can't know how I would really react, and it's because I can't predict which part of my brain has already been short-circuited, or destroyed, or interrupted by the Alzheimer's, so my "normal" coping mechanisms may never be operational again. "Normal" gets to be reinvented many, many times in the lives of people with dementia, and as far as the people with dementia are concerned it's "everyone else" who has the problem with "normal." In their damaged brains, they can't

1

realize that what they say and do isn't normal behavior any more.

Then there's the forgetting. Since one of the "hallmark" signs of Alzheimer's disease is loss of short-term memory, it's entirely possible that I would forget by the next day that I had heard my devastating diagnosis. Yes, I would forget many, many things, but my loved ones (my caregivers) would remember it all every single waking moment of every single day.

When it's all said and done, it's the families and loved ones of people with any type of dementia who experience the greatest emotional suffering because it lasts their entire lifetime. In most instances, as the dementia progresses, the person who has the dementia forgets they have it; they forget that they're forgetting everything. As long as they're not being made to do something they don't want to do, they can be fairly content and can usually live in the moment. When the caregivers can help make those moments calm and happy, the person with dementia will be able to have a quality of life that will not be afforded to those around them. You caregivers and families who are reading this book don't have the luxury of forgetting, and very often, cannot live in the moment because you have to be responsible for this person you love. You have all the responsibility and little or no reward or compensation for your love and dedication aside from knowing that you are making a difference in your loved one's life. That's what you must hold onto: that knowledge, along with every smile you see, every uttered word of love, and every little remembrance that surfaces up out of their damaged brains. It's just not fair, is it? No, it's not fair and it will surely be one of the most challenging jobs you will ever have to do. Nobody comes through dementia as a caregiver unscarred in some emotional, mental, or physical way.

I want you to know that I understand much of what you're experiencing and I know much of what's to come for you. Do not feel as if you're alone in your daily struggles. As long as you hold this book and come with me as we wander through stories of the people with dementia that I have known, worked with, and loved, you will learn from my stories as you are learning every day from your interactions with your loved one with dementia. And it's in that learning that you will find strength to continue. You will find hope that you and your loved one will survive this seemingly never-ending nightmare intact. You will find that you and your loved one can still create and share many, many wonderful moments together. You can still feel the love, help create and share the laughter, and manage the mayhem.

If you are able to allow humor to become a part of your daily routine, you will find that it will be like a best friend who rushes in and rescues you from pain and suffering with a lantern as you struggle along the darkened pathways through dementia. Yes, the pain and the suffering will always be close by, but to choose to find humor in the small things is to choose to move forward with a smile instead of becoming immobile with pain and sadness.

I know it's much easier to say these words than it is to live them, but I also know you will have the rest of your life to grieve the loss of this loved one once they are gone. I beg you to choose not to grieve daily for the small losses you see. I believe this person you love and care for would not wish for you to mourn them before they die, but would instead wish for you to celebrate each small accomplishment with them and to remind them through your example, of what it's like to laugh and to smile.

Nurturing And Humor Are Keys To Calm And Contentment

One of my goals in writing this book is to help educate you, the caregivers, who are the loved ones or friends of the person with dementia, about ways to nurture that person rather than just take care of them. Nurturing is the key that will allow you to learn the best and easiest ways of caring for your loved one. Let me give you an example of what I mean.

You are attempting to fold some laundry while your wife with dementia is pacing. You need to get the laundry finished, and you don't have a lot of time because there are multiple other demands on your time today. Your wife notices the basket and comes over and begins to "help" you fold the clothing, but does so in the wrong way which will contribute to wrinkled clothes and more work for you. If your response to her is something like: *"Martha, let me do this because you're not doing it quite right and I don't have time to do any ironing--you just come over here and watch the birds landing in the bird feeder now and let me finish..."*

You have likely just added to your duties because now Martha is more confused and upset. She is now probably thinking: *"That's my job, and I certainly know how to fold laundry because I've been doing it for years and years, and who are you to tell me to go look at birds when I have work to do? As for ironing, you've never ironed a day in your life, so what are you talking about, and why should I sit and look at birds when I have work to do?"*

Do you see where I'm going with this scenario? Your response has just escalated her confusion and now she's more than likely upset with you. If you were to respond to Martha's attempt at helping in a nurturing manner, you would recognize her need to feel "normal" by doing normal things, her need to feel useful, and to regain her role in your life and in her life. So you would then give Martha what she needs: *"Martha, dear, I thought I would help you with the laundry because you do so much work around here. It's my turn today! Here, you take these to fold and I'll do these* (give her items that won't matter if they wrinkle such as socks or towels). *How about if we take a break after this and just sit and look at all the beautiful birds at the bird feeder?"*

If she happens to fold items incorrectly, let it go, and come back later to refold them at a time when she won't see you. A few wrinkled clothes won't compare to the feeling of satisfaction she receives from doing *her* work. Hearing that you care for her and want to help her will encourage the calm she now feels because you have just nurtured her needs.

If folding clothes is something she enjoys doing, simply keeping a basket of unmatched socks or unfolded towels hidden away to bring out when you see she's restless or looking for something to do, is a wonderful way to frequently nurture those needs.

The same idea can be used for a sink full of "dirty" dishes, or knickknacks that "need" to be dusted every day. As long as the person with dementia seems to enjoy the activity, then you have just enriched their life by reminding them of it. Conversely, if they now no longer seem to enjoy a certain activity, then asking them to do it will only irritate them, which in turn, will complicate your life until they become calm again.

There is another type of nurturing essential for all people. It's nurturing of the soul. To nurture the soul you look for those activities or items that enrich your life and would be missed terribly if they are absent (something like music).

Music is a huge part of many people's lives, and if you can't remember that you love to listen to chamber music while you go about your day, then you will be aware that *something* is missing, and it will contribute to your confusion so you may begin pacing about looking for something to remind you of what's missing. Or, if you can't remember how to turn on the TV to watch a favorite game show (or even that you love to watch the show) you will feel a void and may go looking for something to fill it. If you were a teacher of small children for many, many years and you still love small children, but now rarely see any as you are kept safely at home, you will experience a sense of sadness or loss that you cannot explain. This could be resolved by frequent exposure to children in a daycare or watching them play on a playground.

Focusing on something the person with dementia was passionate about, either in their work, or in their hobbies, and providing frequent exposure to them of that activity (or some version of it) will nourish the soul. This helps that loved one feel a connection to their past; when they and everything around them was normal and familiar.

Familiar becomes forgotten bit by bit, and it's up to the caregiver to provide the reminders of what was familiar and enjoyed. Think for just a moment of what you do when you feel bored. Does your mind start casting about for an activity that you would like to engage in? People with dementia can't necessarily define that what they are feeling is "boredom," but they start to search for something "familiar" and they won't necessarily even know what that is until they see it. The more often you can provide items to reminisce about, or familiar activities to perform, the calmer they will be, and the calmer your life will be. The more they search for some unknown item or activity to fill the voids in their minds, the more often you caregivers will need to run around behind them to do damage control.

Another goal I have for caregivers in the reading of this book is to help you realize that it's a wonderful gift to yourself and to your loved one if you can again allow some humor into your life. Yes, this is a choice you can consciously make every single day. You can take a potentially day-destroying event and turn it into just a little bump in the road along the journey by using your sense of humor and tapping into your loved one's sense of humor.

I have found that people with dementia maintain their sense of humor for a long time and even when they can't verbalize what they're thinking, they often may still have the ability to "get it" when you are using humor. Both you and your loved one will feel a sense of peace and calm when you can introduce humor into your lives every day. Mind you--never laughing *at* the person with dementia, but rather laughing *with* them.

The diagnosis of dementia will be received differently by every person. When caregivers know what this person was like in the past, and they take the time and make the effort to bring out the memories that work best now, nurturing takes place.

Anyone who has lived or worked with people with dementia has wonderful stories to tell about their experiences. And stories always have a lesson to teach those who are willing to learn.

I have several stories in this book about a tiny, feisty woman named Bea, who was a resident in a facility where I worked. I absolutely loved her for her spirit and determination, her sense of right and wrong, and her mischievous little grin. Let me introduce you now to Bea as I begin to tell you some of my stories.

"I Just Say What's On My Mind"

Bea was an 81-year-old woman who only stood about four feet tall. She was always a whirlwind of activity and used to having her orders obeyed or she could escalate into anger or aggression to get her way. Her philosophy seemed to be "if you want something done, you need to just do it yourself because if you wait for someone else to do it, you'll be disappointed." If she encountered a situation where she felt an injustice was being done to anyone, she wouldn't hesitate to speak up to correct it. This was an admirable trait, but when dementia damaged the social barriers in her brain, her inability to reason and act appropriately in social situations resulted in a rather volatile personality.

I recall the time a staff worker came to tell me that Bea had just loudly cursed at her because she had started to vacuum the hallway where Bea had apparently just run the non-electric sweeper broom. Bea felt insulted that this worker would want to vacuum the same floor she had just cleaned and she didn't hesitate to tell her so. The staff worker knew that if she didn't apologize to Bea and plead ignorance, that Bea's anger would escalate to where she would physically attempt to restrain the worker from continuing to vacuum that floor. So the apology was made, and the vacuum was put away until later after Bea had forgotten she had just cleaned the floor.

In this dementia-dedicated assisted-living facility, we were fortunate to have a psychiatrist, Dr. Iminna, come to see his patients there on a monthly basis. I would meet with several of the direct care workers a day in advance of his visits in order to get valuable input on the status of his patients. Dr. Iminna would then meet briefly with the residents in my office to decide if any medications needed to be adjusted.

Dr. Iminna was always extremely polite, meticulous in his manners and with his appearance, and like most psychiatrists, rarely physically touched his patients aside from a handshake. This would be the second time Dr. Iminna had seen Bea, having placed her on a medication the previous month to help take the edge off her volatile behavior.

Bea happened to be in an affectionate, kissing mood that morning; getting and receiving kisses from every staff person she encountered. She would approach everyone she encountered with an upturned face and pursed lips to receive her kisses. So, when I escorted her into my office where Dr. Iminna had just finished hanging his coat on the rack, she saw him and swiftly moved to him, grabbing him around the waist.

"Bend down here!"

"Why do you want me to bend down?"

He was caught off-guard and wasn't sure what her intentions were.

"I want to give you a kiss!

"Oh; thank you, thank you; but we're not going to do that right now. I would like you to just have a seat here on this chair and I'm just going to talk to you for a few minutes. Okay?"

I could tell from the disgruntled look on Bea's face that she was not happy about this as she grudgingly complied. I was silently observing and thought he would have been better off to have just let her give him a kiss on the cheek rather than risk upsetting her. Dr. Immina began his questions to Bea.

"So you remember me, Bea?"

"Of course I remember you!"

"Good! What is my name?"

"Asshole!"

Dr. Iminna and I both gave a surprised laugh.

"Okay. Well, what's your name?"

"Asshole!"

By now Bea had a small grin on her face and she said, *"I'm sorry, but I always just say what's on my mind."*

Bea then settled down and Dr. Iminna went on to chat briefly with her about how she was feeling, what she did for enjoyment, and then he began to write a note in her chart. Bea, who had been sitting quietly and watching him, suddenly jumped off the chair, swiftly moved over to him, grabbed his face between her two hands, and planted a big kiss on his cheek! Dr. Iminna suffered through her attentions and we both had a good laugh about this feisty little woman's determination once I had escorted her out of the office.

Just because a person has dementia, it doesn't mean they will always quickly lose track of a certain thought. Sometimes, like Bea in this situation, they are able to hold onto the thought of what they want, and they may work diligently to get what they want.

This is just one of the many fond memories I have of Bea's time with us in that facility, and you will read more stories about her as you progress through this book. I hope you get a sense of her wonderful spirit and the boldness with which she lived her life.

"My Brains Are Already Gone!"

Eric, a resident in our facility, is sitting in the visitor's chair in my office as he often does. He likes to look out the windows, sometimes makes comments to me, and sometimes dozes off. I'm working quietly at my desk when suddenly I sneeze three times in rapid succession.

I knew I had startled Eric and I said to him: *"Well, Eric, there went the rest of my brains; I might as well go home now."*

Eric laughed and said: *"Well, my brains are already gone!"*

We both felt happier with that brief exchange. And *any* time you can help a person with dementia feel happier, you've done a wonderful thing, and most likely made your job easier as you cared for them.

I used humor frequently with the residents in that facility because I knew that even if they couldn't verbally say the words, if I said something witty or funny, they could often understand the humor of what I said and respond appropriately to it.

When you use humor with a person with dementia, you need to know ahead of time that they will receive it as humor, and if they don't appear to appreciate it or understand it, simply move on to another subject. Care must always be taken to never laugh *at* the person with dementia, but always laugh *with* them.

Laughing at something a person with dementia has done (because they often unintentionally do things that are quite humorous) is fine, only as long as that person isn't going to take offense at it. If they feel that you are belittling them, embarrassing them, or putting them down in any way, they will react the same way you or I would in that case. They would be upset or angry with you, and you have then just made your caretaking job more difficult because they won't want to do anything for you, or with you, if they're upset with you.

"I Might Have To Kick You Out!"

Belle is in the latter stages of her dementia and can present quite a challenge to everyone trying to care for her. She is nothing but skin and bones, and usually sits with her eyes closed and her arms crossed tightly over her chest. She is often cold so getting her to relax her arms to dress, undress, or eat, is futile unless you have made her feel warm and calm. I've learned that Belle loves music, loves to sing, and can be coaxed into relaxing that rigid posture with a gentle touch and music, plus a lot of patience.

I have never claimed to be able to carry a tune, but Belle has never indicated my singing is painful to her, so I often sing to and with her as I care for her. On this particular day, Belle and I are in her 83-degree room listening to the Three Tenors singing and I'm gently exercising her now-relaxed arms. I say to her: *"Belle, wouldn't if be WONDERFUL to be able to just sing out like that, so loud and so free? Oh how I wish I could do that!"*

Belle, with a calm smile on her face and her eyes closed, seems to consider my question seriously for a moment and then says: *"Well, if you did that, I might have to kick you out!"* We share a hearty laugh over that and I apologize for subjecting her to my singing.

Let me tell you the story about when I first met Belle, whom I loved and admired precisely because she

17

could be so feisty with her caregivers. She taught me so much about dementia. Indeed, Belle is the reason I chose to make the subject of dementia my specialty. When I saw what a huge, positive difference I made in her life, something inside me clicked, and I knew working with elders who have dementia was what I wanted, and needed, to be doing.

Belle taught me about how crucial it was to get out of my own reality and get into hers if I wanted every encounter with her to end in a positive way. Unless I could put myself into her mindset, I wouldn't be able to figure out a way to get her to cooperate with anything I needed her to do. The dementia had progressed through her brain to the extent that her physical comfort was her highest priority, and she would literally fight you to get you to stop disturbing her comfort.

Seen from Belle's perspective:

- It didn't matter to her at all if you were disturbing her for her own good (such as changing her wet brief).

- All Belle knew was that she was no longer comfortable, and that someone was physically assaulting her for unknown reasons.

• Her damaged brain would not be able to comprehend *any* explanation you could give her for this intrusion.

When upset, she could no longer say the words "STOP, I DON'T WANT YOU TO DO THAT!" so her only way of communicating that to you would be to become combative.

My initial introduction to Belle was when I was being oriented to the duties required for the night shift position at the skilled facility where Belle lived. I was being shown the ropes by an aide and another nurse-- both of whom had worked at that facility for many years. It was time for rounds and when we entered Belle's room, they flipped the overbed light on high, said loudly, *"Belle, it's time to change your brief,"* and pulled her quilt and blanket off her tightly-curled little body. Belle did what you or I would likely do in the same situation--she screamed and grabbed for the quilt. After all, she had been sound asleep, nice and warm, and suddenly someone turned on the lights and pulled her blankets off. She could only understand that for reasons unknown to her, she was suddenly very uncomfortable so she struck out in the only way she could to get them to stop.

The nurse and the aide were prepared for her reaction and the aide caught and held her wrists while the nurse dodged her kicking feet to get the wet brief off of her. I was standing at Belle's head frantically trying to calm her down, but Belle was enraged. She was screaming, kicking, trying to bite, scratching; anything she could think to do to make them stop. The nurse managed to get the clean brief on her, and they pulled the quilt back up over her, turned the light off, and left the room without another word to her. Belle was left crying as her damaged brain tried to make sense of what had just happened to her. I took a moment to give Belle a few whispered words of comfort and a quick kiss on her forehead, and then had to catch up with my new co-workers. When I reached the hallway, I noticed the aide was rubbing the back of her hand where Belle's nail marks were clearly visible, and I said, *"There has GOT to be a better way to do this!"*

The nurse's response to me was: *"With her? No, she's <u>always</u> like that. You can't do a thing with her. We ought to get combat pay for what we have to put up with from these people."*

"Well, I'm going to try to find a better way because this is just not acceptable!" You can just imagine how that statement immediately endeared me to my new co-workers!

I knew I had to learn more about Belle in order to help take care of her. I learned that she loved music and singing, hated to be cold, and she would respond in a positive way to a gentle, calm, and unhurried approach. Once I learned that, every night I worked I would enter Belle's room alone. I would run the water in the bathroom sink until it was hot to warm the wipes I would use to clean her bottom. I would then ball them tightly in my hand to keep them warm. I would turn the overbed light on low, bend down to her sleeping head and softly sing to her: *"Oh Bell-llle..."*

Every time I did this, she would smile, and without opening her eyes, would sing back: *"Ye-eessss."*

"Hi, Belle. It's Cindy, and I'm here to put a nice dry brief on you." I would be sure to say this with a big smile on my face so it would be conveyed in my tone of voice.

She would usually start to grumble: *"Ohhhh, I don't want to..."*

"Oh, I know you don't want to, Belle, but you know what? I'm going to help you stay nice and warm and I'm going to <u>sing</u> and I want you to sing with me!"

I would begin to sing; it was usually "Amazing Grace," and once I felt her relax and begin to sing with me, I would slowly replace her quilt with the small lap robe I had placed over her for just that reason. I would use the warm wipes on her and when I finished, I would pull the quilt back up over her, kiss her on the forehead, and turn out the light. Belle would be smiling, and she never, ever left her nail marks in my hands. I had just tremendously improved the quality of

Belle's life by taking the time to get into her reality and do what I knew she would respond positively to:

- Respecting her comfort

- Treating her with dignity

- Conveying a feeling of safety with me

- Nurturing and a loving approach

These were all conveyed to Belle in that type of interaction and her responses back to me were always reflective of that.

If I had tried to tell those co-workers they were causing Belle to act with aggression and violence every time they interacted with her, they would have looked at me as if I had grown two heads. After all, "we know how to take care of these people; we've been doing it for years!" I was not "the boss," therefore my input need not be heeded, no matter how effective it appeared. That's a very sad reality in many facilities throughout the United States, but thankfully, it's beginning to change for the better.

I often think fondly of Belle and all she taught me, and hope she is smiling down on me when she sees me interacting appropriately with other elders with dementia--just as she taught me.

"DO IT!! DO IT <u>NOW</u>!!!"

Emma, who had been a teacher of small children for decades, wheeled her wheelchair into my office with a very determined look on her face.

"Good morning, Emma. How are you today?"

"DID YOU DO IT YET?" she demanded in a stern, uncompromising "teacher" voice.

"Did I do what, Emma?"

"YOU KNOW! DID YOU DO IT?"

Because of her dementia she was unable to verbalize what her thoughts were and so resorted to the "you know."

"Umm. No, not yet." Since I have no idea what she's talking about, I decide to say I've not done the deed she's wondering about.

"WELL DO IT! DO IT <u>NOW</u>!"

"Okay. I'll get it done. I promise, just as soon as I finish this!"

This answer satisfies her so she gives me another stern look, nods once, and backs her wheelchair out of my office.

I had no clue as to what she wanted me to do, but she was certain that I did know, so once I reassured her that I would do it, she was satisfied. If she had persisted or stayed to watch me "DO IT" then I would have asked her to help me or show me since "I'm not very good at this." I had to be careful to maintain a serious demeanor throughout this verbal interchange since she was very serious indeed.

Reach For The Sun, Alice

It's 3:40 a.m. and I catch a movement out of the corner of my eye and turn to see Alice slowly ambling down the hallway toward the nurses' station. Her white, wispy hair is pressed flat on one side of her head, and in wild disarray on the other side. She's cold, and has her arms clutched across her chest, no slippers and no housecoat. I rise with a smile and hurry toward her: *"Alice! What woke you up at 3:30 in the morning?"*

"Oh, it's not 3:30, is it? I thought it was time to get up and get ready for work!"

I put my arm around her and slowly begin to turn her back toward her room. *"Yes, it's almost 4 a.m., and you really look cold. Let me help you find something to keep warm."*

"Yes, I'm cold. How do I turn up the heat? But now that I'm up, I might just as well get ready for work. I don't think I'll get back to sleep."

"Oh my! What I wouldn't give some mornings for an extra hour or two of sleep! What time do you need to be ready for work?"

"Oh--I don't know. I guess I'm usually ready by--by--Oh, I don't know. I get ready early."

"I'll tell you what, Alice. You climb back into this nice warm bed. Here's an extra blanket for you, and try to get a little more sleep, and I promise I'll get you up in plenty of time to get ready, PLUS, I'll make sure you get your favorite oatmeal with raisins and brown sugar for breakfast. How does that sound?"

"Well, I don't feel very tired right now. I don't think I'll be able to go back to sleep."

"I understand, and that's fine if you can't. We'll find something to occupy your time if you're up early, but let me put your music on and maybe that will help you. I wouldn't want you to be sleepy all day tomorrow at work."

I tuck her in, put soft, relaxing music on, dim the lights, and sit on the edge of her bed.

"Alice, here's a good way to relax enough to get back to sleep. Tell me about a vacation you once took. Where did you go?"

"Oh--there were so many. You know we always liked to go to Barbados every year. The children just loved it."

"Okay--Alice, close your eyes, and picture yourself on the beach with the children. Feel the hot sun, how your feet feel in the sand, and hear the waves. Can you see all of that?"

Alice smiles and closes her eyes. *"Yes, that sun was pretty hot so I always wore a hat on the beach."*

"What a smart idea that was. Now, I'm going to leave you here to think about Barbados and what a wonderful time you had. Remember the warm sun, and the laughter of the children playing on the beach."

I gently kiss her forehead and quietly leave the room. Alice is snoring softly when I check on her twenty minutes later.

What could I have done if Alice had not been able to go back to sleep or had resisted my redirection back to her bed? Read on.

But What If They Don't Want To Go Back To Sleep?

There were times when Alice or other people with dementia didn't quietly and calmly go back to bed. Disrupted sleep patterns are quite common in dementia and sometimes no matter what you say or do, they just need to stay up and become involved in something.

If Alice had been unable to go back to sleep and came out of her room again, I would have seated her nearby, asked her if she was hungry, and then provided her with a light snack that included a warm beverage. Asking her to fold a basket of towels, or match a basket of socks in order to "help me get my work done" would have kept her occupied for some time. Alice also loved our box of buttons, so I might have asked her to please sort them by size or color for me since "I just never have time to get that done." She loved to be helpful, and she loved it when people would ask her to help them. She would just beam when we hugged her with our profuse thanks for a task well done.

When I attempted to help Alice relax and try to go back to sleep, I was helping her access some good, calming memories, however that can often be fruitless because they will lose the ability to do that as the dementia progresses. But, while they are still quite high-functioning and can clearly recall many events from their past, it usually helps to calm and comfort them.

There is no way to tell if Alice really did continue to visualize her Barbados beach when I left the room, but all of the other comfort measures I took with her contributed to making her feel calm, comfortable, and cared for: which enabled her to relax enough to go back to sleep. The smile, the gentle touch, the concern for her comfort, the promise to help her when she awoke, all helped her feel safe and comfortable. Never underestimate the power of your smile and your gentle touch when you are attempting to help them relax enough to go back to sleep.

When your loved one at home begins to awaken during the night and doesn't seem to be interested in going back to bed, it becomes a huge stressor for you as the caregiver. Ongoing lack of sleep will contribute to just about everything negative you can think of in your life, so it's imperative that you find ways to cope with this common problem. Some things you can do to help facilitate sleep for your loved one include:

- Discourage napping during the day by keeping them as active and engaged as possible in things that interest them.

- Avoid any stressful activities before bedtime such as a bath if they are resistant to having one. Change bath time to the mornings and just do a "wash up" of face, hands, armpits, and peri area before bedtime.

- Try to increase fluid intake early in the day and begin to decrease it or eliminate it a few hours prior to bedtime. It's crucial they get lots of fluids, but not late in the day when it will increase the need to urinate. Toilet them just before bedtime.

- Use soft music and lighting and keep them warm and comfortable prior to bedtime to encourage sleepiness.

- If they don't want to go to bed without you, get dressed for bed and join them until they fall asleep.

- Put a nightlight in the bathroom. One client who had been in the Navy, discovered when he put a red nightlight bulb in his mother's bathroom, she no longer woke up completely when she got up to void. Red lights used inside submarines don't awaken the brain like a white light does, and he credits this simple change with allowing her to simply go back to bed to sleep rather than waking up completely and wondering where she was as she had been doing.

- Exercise is crucial! The more exercise *both* of you have during the day, the better you will *both* sleep during the night. That's only *one* of the many benefits of exercise. Walking is a great way to exercise, and it's sometimes the only way a person with dementia is willing or able to "exercise." Care must be taken to not overdo it though because of the risk of fatigue and falling, not to mention becoming irritated at being asked to do something they may not want to do.

If nothing you try seems to work, and you are losing a lot of sleep trying to keep tabs on your loved one, sometimes a minimal dose of a sleep aid for your loved one (prescribed by the doctor) can help them sleep better. Periodically check to see if they can be weaned off this medication as their dementia progresses since all medications have side effects and if they can sleep without it, that's the preferred way.

Another option, although an expensive one, is to have caregivers come in to sit with your loved one overnight. I also know of at least two large families who created a sleep-over schedule for the children of the person with dementia so their parent was never alone at night. Because there were five or more children living nearby to share this load, nobody got burned out and they saved a lot of money.

When it's all said and done, the person with dementia will suffer a LOT less than you will from an ongoing lack of sleep. So I urge you to become creative in finding ways to get plenty of sleep in order to continue caring for this loved one.

Redirecting Ella Mae's Thoughts

It was a very long time ago, shortly after I graduated from practical nursing school, that I was asked to assist with companion care for an elderly woman with dementia who was living in a nursing facility. I knew virtually nothing about how to interact with people with dementia at that time since little was taught in nursing school, aside from the horrible, incorrect belief that people with dementia should <u>always</u> be re-oriented. It just never seemed right to me to continually try to force a person to change their mind about something of relative insignificance when it was clearly upsetting them and frustrating to me. So here I was, this young, inexperienced, newly graduated practical nurse going in to visit with a sweet and confused elderly lady several times a week.

Ella Mae was a thin, petite woman who always had her gray/white hair put up in a small bun on top of her head. She was usually pretty calm and content, but sometimes for reasons she was unable to verbalize, she would begin to get agitated or she would start to cry. She had a bookshelf in her room containing some of her treasures and among them were two crystal birds that would easily fit into her small hands. One of them was completely blue and the other was completely red. They were delicately shaped handblown glass, and when the sun touched them they became beautiful little points of light in her room. I quickly learned that presenting one of these birds to her would bring a smile of joy to her face and she would always relax and become calm again. I don't believe the term "redirecting" was even being used in the context of dementia at that time, but that was exactly what I was doing. In a gentle, nonconfrontational way, I redirected whatever negative thoughts she was having by giving her a favorite object to focus on. For some people, bringing up a favorite topic or memory will redirect their agitation back to a calm state. People with dementia can only focus their damaged brains on one thing at a time, and this is what happened to work well with Ella Mae.

She didn't seem to know the glass birds belonged to her, and was always surprised and delighted to see them. I would tell her these birds belonged to her and she always reacted with delight, as if I had just given her a beautiful gift. She would gently caress one of them in her soft, pale hands and seemed to favor the red bird while I always felt the blue bird was more beautiful. I would chat on about how lovely they were, and she would agree by nodding or simply saying "yes" with a smile since her dementia had claimed many of her words.

I always enjoyed my time with Ella Mae and was saddened one day when her daughter called to tell me Ella Mae had passed on the previous night. As I reminisced with Mae Lynn about her mother and how those glass birds always brought a smile of joy to her face, Mae Lynn graciously asked me if I wished to have one of them to remember her mother. I chose the blue bird and almost thirty years later, every time I look at it, I can't help but reflect the memory of that sweet woman's smile with one of my own.

A Worthy Goal

As in the previous story with Ella Mae, learning how to successfully redirect a person with dementia is just the beginning of the communication tools caregivers and friends must master in order to achieve a good quality of life for that person. Once this skill is mastered, the lives of the caregivers will also be enhanced because the number of crises they must deal with will decrease.

Caregivers of people suffering with dementia continually strive to maintain or improve the health, happiness, safety, and dignity of the dementia sufferer. This is a worthy goal to pursue, whether you are dealing with a friend, a family member, or are in a professional nurse-patient relationship. In order to achieve the goal, it is essential that the caregivers change the way they are interacting with this person with dementia. You are the one who has to do all the changing in terms of approach and attitude because this person with dementia cannot. Their damaged brains can no longer be held responsible for what they're saying and doing, and *they cannot change.* If you want to strive to meet this worthy goal, as well as decrease the number of crises happening daily, then you need to change in your every interaction with them. It's definitely not easy to make any of those changes in yourself or in the way you interact with this person, there isn't much about any aspect of dementia that is easy, but it's crucial.

When you're caring for a loved one with dementia at home you may feel as if you're just struggling to get through the next hour or day because you just don't know what will hit you next. You don't even know what questions to ask if you do ask for help. Every family caregiver has felt as if their lives have become a series of crises with this loved one with dementia. You emerge from one crisis, perhaps unscathed, perhaps with wounds, and try to make life normal again while wondering when and how the next crisis will hit. Maybe some of you don't think about that at all; maybe you just know on some level there will be a crisis, and when that happens you will handle that one, and the one after that, and the one after that; and I think that's not such a bad way to live. It is not good to "obsess" about the problems one encounters in life, let alone about things that haven't happened yet. Perhaps that is what the old adage "Don't borrow trouble" means. In the constant up and down world of the caregiver, a better way to live is to think less about the daily "crises" and focus more on what went right that day, and how can we have more "right" days? I don't mean that you shouldn't have plans for certain crises, because the more aware and prepared you are for them, the better the outcome. Being able to see an incident such as finding the milk in the kitchen cupboard as just a minor bump in the day rather than as a crisis, will help you keep your stress level lower.

A "crisis" is more about really big issues such as wandering away and getting lost, driving and hurting someone, or leaving the stove burner on and causing a fire. You should definitely look at those potential crises and make plans ahead of time rather than just hope they won't ever happen. Having your loved one carry identification, and installing locks on the doors, disabling the car, and removing the burner dials or installing a kill switch on the stove are all steps you may take in your "plan" for those types of crises.

As you may have already discovered in communicating with your loved one with dementia, even a simple conversation can be upsetting and cause an angry or frustrated eruption. If you react to those emotions in a like manner, you are soon involved in a shouting match with your loved one: a match you will never win. But even shouting matches have a lesson to teach you so you can plan for what to say, and how to react the next time that happens, what to say and what to do so the shouting part happens less frequently. As frustrating and scary as it may be, if you want to have less turmoil in interactions with your loved one, you are the one who has to do the changing because your loved one no longer can.

The following story about Janice and Kyle shows how both their lives changed for the better once Kyle was able to change the way he interacted with his wife.

Facing The Painful Truth

Janice and Kyle's story is very typical of what many families are experiencing. It illustrates how the family confronts the diagnosis and learns how to live with a loved one with dementia.

In the sixty-two years of their marriage, Janice had always been the one to pay the bills, keep the checkbook, and run the household. She was a small, thin woman who liked to be active throughout the day with various projects. She spent much of her time cleaning her house, but lately it seemed that she was having difficulty completing the tasks she had started, and she was often frustrated by that.

Kyle, Janice's husband, was a retired factory worker whose voice on the phone sounded very tired and defeated, as if he was dreading speaking every word about his situation to me.

The first time Kyle really acknowledged something was truly wrong with Janice was when she was handicapped due to a foot injury when she had stumbled and fallen. On this day, Janice had handed Kyle a large stack of bills to be mailed and as he walked out to the mailbox he idly leafed through the envelopes. Much to his dismay he found two envelopes addressed to the electric company, there were several envelopes to companies and charities he had never heard of before, and there was no envelope to the bank for the car payment he knew should have been there.

"That's when I just sat down on the curb and knew in my heart that I had to finally admit something was terribly wrong here."

He had opened the electric bills and one of them was accompanied by a check dated two months in the future, and the other was a late payment notice and had no check at all with it.

Kyle sat out there on that curb in the cold December wind for a long time as all the memories came back to him of the friends and relatives who had been dropping hints about Janice's forgetfulness. He also recalled how he had brushed off those hints and had explained them away because it was just too painful to consider the reasons.

"She's been a little under the weather lately but she just won't go to the doctor. She says she just needs to get more rest. She's got a lot on her mind right now with the kids coming home for Christmas. Every time I try to tell her she's done something the wrong way or that she needs to see the doctor, she just blows up at me and I almost feel like I'm back in the war again. She says I don't love her anymore when I try to tell her she's wrong and that just about breaks my heart."

As Kyle told me this sad story I could hear a catch in his voice, and I felt the tears forming in my own eyes as I began to understand the pain he was going through. After sixty-two years of marriage, he was beginning to see disturbing changes in his beloved wife and he was now forced to admit her decline to himself. Kyle loved his wife and he was bewildered by her accusations and her actions, and now he seemed frozen by grief, fear, and sadness and had no idea of what steps to take next.

Kyle had not yet said anything about his fears to their two adult children, both of whom would be coming home for Christmas in just a few weeks.

"I don't want to worry them when I don't know myself what's wrong. Maybe it's just something little that the doctor can fix with some medicine and she'll be fine, so I don't want to get them all worried for nothing."

I asked Kyle a lot of questions that would tell me more about Janice's short-term memory abilities, and reassured him that it's quite normal for families to deny what they are seeing for some time until it can no longer be denied. What was most important was that he was now taking action to identify and solve the problems.

"Well, once I admitted to myself that she was having problems, I saw where she covers up a lot of

things she forgets, like appointments, or if she talks to someone on the phone she seems to forget a lot of those calls."

Kyle remembered just last week one day when Janice had left the kitchen after supper at his request to watch a television special with him, and they had then gone to bed. The next morning when Janice came into the kitchen and found dirty pots and pans from the night before, she had snapped at Kyle for never helping her out around the house. During the entire sixty-two years of their marriage Janice had always declined any help in her kitchen and certainly had never left dirty dishes overnight. He also recalled how she never wanted to go grocery shopping alone anymore. She said she just couldn't handle all those bags by herself, and now that he was thinking about it, she never shopped with a grocery list any more. She always said she had forgotten it and the grocery shopping was now accomplished by moving slowly through all the aisles looking at everything and taking twice as long.

Kyle had returned to the house with the bills and when he asked to see the checkbook, Janice had become very angry and shouted at him that from then on he could just do it all himself. She refused to listen as he tried to show her the errors in the checkbook and had locked herself in the bedroom and cried for a long time. Still, she adamantly refused to go to the doctor for a check-up.

Kyle was calling me for advice on how he could convince her to go to the doctor, or just what he should do next. I told him I thought it sounded like Janice was experiencing some short- term memory loss, and that she was aware of the problem to some extent, thus the "blow-ups" when he attempted to point out her errors. She was beginning to lose control in several areas of her life and she was understandably afraid of what might be happening. I cautioned him that short-term memory loss does not necessarily mean Alzheimer's, and that she truly did need to be seen by her doctor so he could rule out a lot of other things that could be causing it, things that could be cured. Among other things, the doctor would check her vitamin B12 level, thyroid function, blood sugar, and her urine. He might also order a scan of her brain. The challenges now were how to convince her to go to the doctor for those tests, as well as how to keep her more calm and content.

It was imperative that Kyle stop trying to always convince Janice she had done things wrong. He agreed that every time he did that, Janice would "blow up." Kyle needed to begin taking the blame, if needed, for anything that went awry in order to help Janice stay calm.

"If Janice yells at you for not helping around the house because she's forgotten to clear the dishes, then simply apologize to her, tell her you'll try to do better, and start helping. You'll avoid that blow-up that you would normally have had when she perceived it was

her own forgetfulness causing the problem. Janice is never going to be convinced by you that the problem lies with her, so stop trying to convince her. Brush off the lapses in memory, or say 'I'm sorry, I must have forgotten to tell you about that appointment. I'll write it down next time.' The calmer you can make Janice's life, the calmer your life will be."

It was crucial to have Kyle see that point, but it would be exceedingly difficult for him to change, as it is for anyone in a marriage of many years to do. People develop a unique style of interacting and communicating with each other, and when asked to suddenly and completely change that style, will usually have a lot of trouble doing so. I told Kyle that humor could help in some instances, especially if Janice had a good sense of humor, which he said she often did. If she said she "forgot" the grocery list again, rather than reinforce her negative feelings and become upset himself, he could choose to say with a smile something like: *"Well, we'll just have a grand adventure today in the store and pick out anything we like!"*

Another important thing Kyle could do was try to continually remind Janice that he loved her and that he needed her. If she was lashing out at him because she was afraid she was losing control of her abilities, then she might possibly feel she would become a burden to him if she couldn't continue to do all of the things she had done their entire married life; that Kyle wouldn't love her as before because he wouldn't "need" her anymore. When she prepared a meal, simply saying something like: *"Honey, that was great! You take such good care of me all the time and I just don't tell you often enough how much I love and appreciate you for it."*

Maybe Janice could articulate some of her fears, and maybe she couldn't, but she could certainly feel rejected, useless, and incompetent when she was being accused by Kyle of doing something wrong. I asked Kyle to try to imagine how he would feel if one day he couldn't remember how to use the telephone when he wanted to make a call that he used to make without even thinking about how to do it. He agreed that he would feel afraid, as well as defensive. He would feel the need to cover it up, to explain it away, and he would probably get angry if Janice insisted he get himself to the doctor immediately. Now I felt Kyle was beginning to see why Janice reacted to him as she had, and he seemed to feel he would be able to stop pointing out her mistakes and upsetting her by remembering to employ the following tips:

- Ignoring the mistakes and not pointing them out.

- Using humor to explain or justify a mistake.

- Taking the blame for negative outcomes.

All of these actions would help Janice cope better with her fears, and would result in her being calmer, which in turn would make Kyle's life calmer.

I offered Kyle several suggestions for getting Janice to her doctor. *"Schedule an appointment for both of you at the same time, and make a deal with Janice that you will get your problem checked out if she would go just to see if her vitamins (which she firmly believed was something they needed to be taking every day) were still appropriate."*

Kyle could "create" a physical problem for himself or he could just be following up on an existing one he might already have. It would be important for him to assure Janice that it was nothing out of the ordinary for both of them to get checked out, and that he would be with her the entire time if she wished. Janice's need to have Kyle accompany her to the grocery store indicated she was pretty uncomfortable being alone in public places, and would likely feel better if he assured her he would stay with her. It would also be important for Kyle to call the doctor's office ahead of time to tell them his fears, and to caution them not to frighten her off with talk of a big "Alzheimer's work-up" and to be aware of her reluctance to even be there.

"Another option, Kyle, would be to sit down with Janice at a time when she's calm, hold her hands and make eye contact with her. In a gentle, calm voice tell her she's the love of your life, that you could never

imagine life without her, and that you want her to stay with you for the next fifty years. When she's processed that, then tell her that because you love her so much, you want her to always be in the best of health, which means she needs to be seen regularly by the doctor, and it is time to schedule an appointment now because it has been over a year since her last visit."

Again, notifying the doctor's office ahead of time regarding concerns about her memory lapses would be important. If Janice still refused, I asked Kyle if he felt either or both of the children could persuade her. Kyle said Janice had a "really good relationship" with their daughter, but he felt their daughter was just too "flighty" to be of much help in keeping Janice calm, and didn't think their son would be able to convince her either, so that was not an option.

Kyle wondered if they should just tell Janice that they suspected a memory problem and that she had no choice but to go for a check-up. An "intervention" by loved ones in a confrontational manner by sitting the person with dementia down and telling them why they need to see the doctor, reassuring them they're loved, and demanding that they be seen (such as is done with alcoholics and drug addicts) may result in tearful acquiescence, but if the person then forgets about the entire intervention by the time the appointment comes around, it's of little value. I suspected that would be the outcome of such a meeting with this family. Since the goal here was to get Janice to the doctor for a work-up, and also to keep her as calm and happy as possible, I told Kyle about another option.

"Kyle, since you know Janice's short-term memory seems to be affected right now, that means that it's likely she won't remember tomorrow something you tell her today." Kyle agreed with that.

"If your goal is to keep Janice as calm and happy as possible, and get her into the doctor's office, then another option would be to just schedule the appointments--for both of you, or just for her-- whichever you believe she would more readily accept-- to not tell Janice in advance anything about it since she would be likely to forget anyway, and just show up at the office at the appointed time. She would likely recognize the place, and you could then, in a calm and unhurried manner, say: 'Oh my gosh! Don't tell me I forgot to tell you about this! Yes--because we're overdue for check-ups, and I've been having this little problem, I went ahead and scheduled these appointments!' The entire time you're explaining this, you are calmly getting out of the car and assisting her to exit the car and head into the office, 'I'm so sorry I forgot to tell you. We're right on time now, so we can't cancel them. They'll just charge us anyway if we don't go now. Come on, honey, I'll stay with you during your appointment if you want me to. Just don't you tell the doctor how terribly I've messed this up!' Keep holding her hand or arm and keep yourself calm, using humor if it's helping

to keep her calm. 'I swear I must be getting senile these days. I've probably forgotten to zip my zipper too!'"

"If Janice's social graces are intact, my guess is that she won't want to cause a scene in the office, and will go along with you. Once you're settled in the waiting room just chitchat about whatever she will listen to and remain calm. Don't jump in with answers if she can't appropriately answer the nurse or doctor's questions, just maintain that calm and reassuring presence at her side. If you've told the doctor's office in advance of your concern about memory loss, they should be discreet about the language they use to describe what they're doing and why."

It was important for Kyle to remain calm during the entire scenario because Janice would be taking her cues from him. She would likely respond with apprehension, possibly anger, and the calmer he could remain, the more it would help him accomplish the goals. Knowing it would be embarrassing for Janice to go through the "memory test," because she would likely miss a number of the questions, I told Kyle what I would often say to people to help calm them before I administered the memory test in the physician's office where I had worked.

"This is a little test we give to all of our patients when they reach a 'certain age' and then we will give it to you every year hereafter. Don't worry if you miss some of the questions, because if you do miss a few,

then that tells us that we need to be checking to see if your medications (or vitamins) are still working well for you."

If they were unable to accurately count backwards from one hundred, I would joke that I would probably need to use fingers and toes to do that since math was never my favorite subject. I would continually be trying to keep that person in the most relaxed and compliant mood possible. I would also be sure to accompany the person with dementia to another area (whether under the pretense of going through the list of meds or asking them questions about their spouse) and stay with them while giving the doctor time to talk privately with the spouse. I told Kyle he would need to have time to process the information from the doctor in order to make a decision about more tests and getting a diagnosis, thus the private conversation.

Janice would likely accept an explanation from the doctor that the exam and testing today showed she was having "just a little bit of a memory problem," and since there are so many reasons that could be happening (without mentioning Alzheimer's or dementia), he wanted to draw some blood, or take some scans, in order see if it was caused by something such as not enough vitamin B12, or her thyroid gland acting up.

If Janice expressed anger to Kyle after the appointment, he would need to again apologize profusely for forgetting to tell her, maybe offer to take her to dinner, or say whatever he needed to help her become calm again. He could say something like: *"But I'm glad we're done with that now and that we're both in pretty good shape for such old folks..."* This would help reassure Janice that it was over and that they didn't tell her anything was terribly wrong with her. Using that expression "a little memory problem" would come in handy when it came time for further testing or even a new medication.

Kyle felt the last option would probably be the one he had to go with, and armed with a new awareness of just how his mood and the words he chose to use affected Janice's actions, he felt he could get through it successfully.

Another very important suggestion I gave to Kyle was to begin the process of acquiring a durable healthcare power of attorney for Janice so that he, or whomever she chose, would have the authority to make healthcare decisions for her if needed. Again, going through the same process himself would reassure Janice that this was a normal thing that needed to be done, and not a reflection on her abilities in any way. Kyle later reported to me that Janice had chosen him and her son as powers of attorney, and because she was quite interested in who he would choose, Kyle chose Janice and their son, knowing that the son would have full power of attorney if Janice were unable to act in that capacity. He reported that Janice was quite pleased to see that in the legal document because it told her she was still valued and trusted by her husband.

It turned out pretty much as we had anticipated with Janice at the doctor's office. She had been reluctant to get out of the car until a woman they knew approached with a small baby, and as Kyle made a fuss over the baby, Janice had exited the car to see the baby. She was reluctant to cause a scene in the office, so she complied with Kyle and the testing, and after all the lab tests and the CT scan, Janice was found to be in the early to middle stages of Alzheimer's. Kyle was told in private of the diagnosis, and elected to tell his children by phone before they arrived for the holiday, so they would have some time to process the information, and also to change their expectations of what the holiday would be like. They decided to tell Janice of the diagnosis once they were all together so they could continually reassure her of their love and support.

Janice took the news surprisingly well with only a small flare of anger at the beginning. Kyle reported "*it was almost as if she was relieved that she didn't have to wonder anymore.*" Janice was able to make some end-of-life decisions with her family present during that holiday which relieved them of that responsibility, and comforted them that they would be doing exactly what she wanted at the end of her life. She was even able to tell Kyle, "rather emphatically," that if the time came when she couldn't take care of herself, that he should take her "somewhere close by where other people could help" take care of her. What a blessing that was for Kyle and his children when Janice suffered a fractured hip about a year later and then required admission to a nearby nursing home. The memory of Janice's insistence that she be placed in a facility if that time came made that extremely difficult time just a bit easier for them to bear.

We tend to believe that once people receive a diagnosis of some type of dementia, they have now become mentally unable to make any appropriate healthcare decisions for themselves. People in the early stages can still make competent healthcare decisions, and I know from my many years of experience that especially in the early stages, and even into the middle stages for some people, there can be times when it's as if the clouds part in the brain, and they become lucid for very short periods of time. Those are the bittersweet times for families when they welcome that recognition back, that brief ability to suddenly make sense before it's gone again.

As you have seen in this story about Janice and Kyle, it's especially difficult for a spouse to change the way they have been interacting with their loved one. After all, in your situation, the two of you have been responding to one another in a certain pattern for your entire married life, but now you must change that pattern. Here are some of the most crucial things I want you to always remember from reading this book:

•It will be _your_ actions and reactions in any situation that will determine the outcome of that situation with a person with dementia.

•When you can change your actions and reactions to become nonconfrontational or non-blaming, the stresses you both feel will be greatly lessened.

Holiday Pins and Needles

This story is about some of the many struggles a daughter whose mother with Alzheimer's experienced in the challenging early stages of the disease. Lynette called me and explained her situation: *"My mother is in the early stages of Alzheimer's and lives at home with my father. The problem I am faced with is that every holiday my family and I spend a week with my parents in their home. My mother was always such a calm and happy person, but lately when I speak to her on the phone, she's very quick to argue with things I say, becomes angry, and sometimes slams the phone down. My father makes excuses for her such as 'she's just tired,' or 'you know she's having a hard time.' I can't spend the entire holiday on pins and needles or have my two young sons subjected to her angry tirades every day. I need some suggestions as to how I might handle this."*

This was the problem Lynette initially contacted me about, but I could see that as with any dilemma in a relationship with another person, there were several other huge questions being asked at the same time. The other questions I heard being asked included:

* *"Why is Mom so unhappy now and what can we do about it?"*

- *"Why does she treat me this way? Doesn't she love me anymore? Or is it that she's forgetting that I'm her only daughter?"*

- *"Why doesn't Dad ever take my side in this and help me find a way to make Mom happy and calm again?"*

- *"Am I a bad daughter for not wanting to see my family on the holiday?"*

- *"Have we lost Mom forever to Alzheimer's?"*

I reassured Lynette that the personality changes, mood swings, and anxiety could all be part of Alzheimer's disease, and the most important thing for Lynette and her entire family to realize was that her mom's ability to sort out and cope with stimulus of any kind was permanently altered. Mom *could* *not* change the way she was reacting, so it would be up to everyone around her to change the way they approached her or responded to her. For instance, if Mom thought it was Tuesday instead of Saturday, let her be right and drop the subject. Take the blame for getting everything wrong: *"Oh, I'm sorry, I must have gotten my days mixed up. Let's go to the kitchen now and..."*

The family should save any re-orienting to reality or demanding they are right for those instances when there is a danger such as if she decided to drive the car. Even in that case, it would be extremely important to preserve her dignity with something like: *"Mom, I'm going to treat you like a queen today, and queens never drive themselves anywhere. Billy would like you to point out some of the sights as we drive past, so you just sit here in the back with your grandson and enjoy the ride like the queen you are today."*

I told Lynette that the "pins and needles" would probably always be there to some extent with the family since you can never be sure of what a person with dementia is thinking, or how they might respond in any given circumstance. I suggested to Lynette that to minimize everyone's stress, it might be better if she and her family stayed elsewhere nearby her parent's home, and just visited with them daily. To suddenly force her mother to live with two small children and two more adults would be asking for too much since it would quickly overwhelm her limited abilities to cope. Limiting the time they spent with her mom would avoid much of that overstimulation and thus, the outbursts that would undoubtedly follow.

I also suggested they keep distractions on hand for her mother. Keeping items such as a family photo album or holiday decorations out in the open for easy access would provide "safe" topics since she could reminisce about whatever it was that she remembered about them. They needed to avoid pointing to a picture and asking "Do you remember who this is?" because if she didn't recall who it was, it would only frustrate or embarrass her, either of which could lead to her becoming angry. Instead, giving her hints such as "I remember when Dad took this picture of me and my puppy. I think I may have been around five years old..." may help her remember, and if she doesn't seem to recall, then simply move on to the next picture. When she successfully recalls a memory, keeping her on that subject for as long as she enjoys talking about it would help her feel content and calm.

It was important that Lynette tell her children in advance something to the effect that "*Grandma won't be able to remember everything, and that's okay, but we must try to help her be happy. We won't be asking her if she remembers things, instead we'll just give her the answers ahead of time, so she doesn't get so tired and upset.*" It would be important for Lynette and her family to continually be alert for signs that her mother was becoming tired or frustrated, and take immediate steps to alleviate that. If the children took naps, might there be a way to incorporate that into a nap for Grandma also?

It was also important for Lynette's father to take her mother to their family physician (notifying the office in advance of her mood swings) to see if a very small dose of a medication might help to take the edge off her anxiety, or to possibly diagnose and treat a clinical depression.

To address those unspoken questions I felt Lynette was asking in the beginning, I had written them down and addressed them near the end of our conversation in the following way:

•Why is Mom so unhappy now and what can we do about it?

"Lynette, you and your family must realize that just about every thought that comes into your mother's mind now can cause her more confusion, which increases her anxiety and can trigger anger. An example might be, if you and your mother are sitting and quietly talking and the phone suddenly rings beside her. That could trigger sudden anxiety or anger in her because her damaged brain may not quickly be able to figure out what that sudden, loud, irritating noise is and she may not remember how to stop it, so she may slap at the phone just to get it to stop the noise which is confusing her. She has lost her reference points in her mind that instantly tell her what that noise is, why she hears the noise, and that if she simply picks up the receiver, the noise will stop and she can talk to someone who is calling her. Without those reference points, it's just a sudden, loud, irritating noise to be stopped."

"Without dwelling on what she has lost, it's important to focus on what she has left and give her every opportunity to 'remember' and use those memories that still make sense to her. The more she can make sense of what is being said or done, or what she says or does, the calmer and happier she will be. In

the telephone example, if I saw that it was upsetting her, I would calmly walk over, pick up the receiver to stop the noise, briefly hold my hand over the receiver while I smile at her and say something like: 'These telephones are so terribly loud and annoying, aren't they, Mom? It always scares me when they ring right beside me. I almost jumped out of my skin! Excuse me just a minute, Mom, while I ask who is calling.' By giving her clues as to what the noise is, validating her feelings by agreeing that it is a scary thing and she's right to be upset, and also treating her with respect, you would help to quickly calm her anxiety."

•Why is Mom treating me this way? Doesn't she love me anymore, or is she forgetting that I'm her only daughter?

"It's extremely important, Lynette, for you and your family to not take it personally when your mom forgets or when she lashes out in anger or in fear. This is not the way your mom would act or talk or treat people she loved if she were still 'in her right mind.' This is a very sad reality of dementia. It's also a sad reality that when we're frustrated and upset, sometimes we take it out on the people closest to us even if we don't have dementia. Your mother's love for her family is still there inside her brain, but now many of the pathways to access those memories have been disrupted. When the influx of stimuli is bombarding her damaged brain, it's all she can do to just try and make sense of what was just said, and she can't access those loving feelings

and thoughts because her brain can't find them quickly enough. Given enough time and the 'right' words and body language, at this point in your mom's dementia, she could likely access her love for her family and be able to express those feelings, but not when she's frustrated, confused, or angry. People with dementia can only focus on one thing at a time which leaves no room for considering other people's feelings."

"Lynette, it's important that you try not to take these outbursts personally. I know that it hurts you deeply to have your mother say untrue things to you in an angry tone. Even if you can tell yourself 'it's the dementia talking,' it still hurts and you need to acknowledge that and then try to just let it go."

"For example, let's say you show up at the house before the holidays and your mother takes one look at you and says in an annoyed tone of voice, 'Why didn't you tell me you were coming to visit?' when you know you had discussed it the day before with her on the phone. Obviously she's not happy about your 'surprise' visit and her overriding thought may be 'Oh no! Here are a bunch of people who will expect me to have a clean house and cook meals for them. It's just too much for me! What will I do?' Because she's having this negative thought and feeling pressured to do something she doesn't feel up to, she's not able to get past these feelings to access the joy at seeing her daughter and her family standing before her. She's unable to find that pathway in her brain because right at this

moment she's feeling stressed by whatever thought is dominant. Nor is she able to access the area of her brain that contains the social graces that say it's more polite to hide your frustration at surprise visitors and welcome them in with open arms and smiles. So she reacts in the only way she can at this time, with the feelings that are closest to the surface."

"Lynette, suppose your reaction to her statement is to immediately look sad, lose your smile of joy, and say something like, 'But Mom, we just talked about it yesterday, and you said you were thrilled that we were coming today!' That's a normal response to a normal situation, but now that your mother has dementia, normal doesn't count for anything anymore. Since your brain is still quite agile, you can immediately perceive that she's upset, she obviously doesn't recall your phone conversation from yesterday. No amount of reorienting will work just now, and it's *your* reaction that will determine how this conversation will end. So without missing a beat, you simply take her hand, change your smile into an apologetic look, and say something like: 'Mom, I'm so sorry! I thought I had called you to tell you we were coming. I'm just mortified that I could forget something like that. Sometimes I think having children has made my brain go soft. We're only here for a few hours and I'm so happy to see you again. I've missed you terribly, Mom. I'm sorry I forgot to call you. Can you forgive me?'"

"Give her a hug and possibly say: 'The boys have missed their favorite grandma, too!' If you detect any softening of her attitude, you know you've managed to get past her initial defenses and you can add something like, 'Mom, I want to give you the gift of relaxation tonight, so I'm going to ask that you sit down and enjoy your grandsons and I'll make your favorite dinner. It's the least I can do to make up for my mistake!'"

"By accurately guessing at what she might be thinking and why, you can defuse her feelings of anxiety and get her to focus on some positive thoughts, but you need to avoid the temptation to re-orient or remind her because the damage in her brain won't allow her to see or admit mistakes easily."

•Why doesn't Dad take my side and help me find a way to make Mom happy and calm again?

"Using the same scenario I just mentioned, what if your response to your mother's remark had been to remind her that you did tell her on the phone yesterday, and then you looked at your father for affirmation and asked him to remind your mother of that. Stop and think for just a moment what might result from that. You have just told your mother she's got it all wrong and you're right. She has forgotten this important event, and that her husband is taking your side and not supporting her when she clearly does not recall being told! Why on earth would she forget such an important phone conversation and why isn't her

husband helping her out here? Her frown would likely deepen, and she would immediately go into a more defensive mode, only now she would be truly alone because she wouldn't be able to count on her husband for any support. So your mother would become more upset, and your father would be placed right in the middle with no way to answer you without upsetting someone. That is a difficult position for anyone to be in. In this instance, the smart response would be to put his arm around his wife and say something like: 'You know, Lynette, I don't recall that phone conversation either--but let's not haggle over that. You're here now, and you look as beautiful as your mother did when she was your age! Don't you think she looks just as beautiful as you did when we first met, dear?'"

"He would know that he's risking upsetting you with this 'therapeutic fib' of not recalling the phone call, but he also knows that you can get over your bad mood much easier than his wife can."

"Your father is also under a tremendous amount of stress and experiencing those same pins and needles that you do around your mother. As she struggles every day to make sense of her confusing thoughts, he struggles every day to help her find some peace within that ocean of confusion. While he's trying to help her make sense of her world, he's also being forced to watch the woman he loves and the mother of his children die one brain cell at a time. His stress level is huge and he must take good care of his own physical and mental

well-being because it's not at all unusual for the caregiver of a person with dementia to die first due to the stress and the tendency to ignore their own health. So please urge your father to consider some of the following options:

•In-home assistance, possibly disguised as part-time cleaning help.

•Friends to come in to be with your mother so he can get out of the house for awhile on a regular basis.

•Joining a local support group could provide invaluable help to him in many different ways, so please encourage him to do that. I urge you to do that as well. Just being able to talk to other people who are experiencing many of the same feelings and challenges could greatly reduce your anxiety and stress levels. You would also hear many great caregiver tips in these groups, all of which would contribute to reducing the stress you experience in these very troubling times with your mom."

I then addressed Lynette's next concern.

•Am I a bad daughter for not wanting to see my family for the holiday?

"Lynette, please try to avoid feeling guilty about questioning if you should even be going to your parents' home for the holidays. We all know that the holidays

themselves add extra stress to everyone's life and when a loved one has dementia, those holiday stresses can become breaking points in so many ways."

"Family holiday traditions can either be a source of comfort for a person with dementia, or they can be a source of increased confusion and chaos for them. Based on what you've told me about your mother's current state, I would guess that her reactions would fall more into the latter category."

"Maybe it's time for you and your husband to start new holiday traditions with your children that could still include your parents, but just wouldn't involve them for the entire week. Would spending just a day or two alone with your parents before or after the holidays be an option? I would urge you to brainstorm with your father and your husband on ways to not only decrease the stress on all of you during the holidays, but also discuss ways to minimize overstimulating your mom while still helping all of you enjoy some quality time together."

•Have we lost Mom forever to Alzheimer's?

"Alzheimer's may have taken many of your mother's memories away, but she still has the ability to enjoy life and experience happy times with her loved ones. The opportunities are also there for you and your family to create some wonderful holiday memories involving her. Keeping every interaction with your

mom short and simple and remaining positive and upbeat will minimize overstimulating her. Taking every opportunity to give her hugs and to tell her how much she means to you will reassure your mom that at this moment in time, all is well with her and she is loved. She will then be more able to simply relax and enjoy your company."

"As I mentioned before, if your mom is suffering from constant anxiety or depression, then a consult with her doctor is needed to determine if a low dose of an anti-depressant can help with that."

"Your mom is still present and needing more love and attention than ever before. It will be a continuing, but not insurmountable challenge for you and your family to find ways to access those memories your mom has left. Don't lose sight of the fact that even when you can't help her remember, she is still someone you love and cherish, and when your every response to her comes from that nurturing thought, she will benefit in ways you can never know."

"He's Selling All My Fur Coats!"

This story illustrates a few of the many challenges spouses face in the early stages when dementia begins to change just about every aspect of their loved one, and their world becomes a daily dance on eggshells just to get through that day.

The elderly woman on the phone was calling me because she was told by her physician that she must.

"My doctor told me that my health is going downhill because my husband has dementia, and I guess I need some help to figure out how to handle it better."

"Mrs. Samson, can you tell me what your home situation is like right now?"

"Well, it's just me and my husband, Tom, here in the house. We've been married for fifty-eight years and now he's got some kind of dementia and I have to figure out how to take care of him. I'm not going to put him in a home because that would just kill both of us, and besides, he insists he doesn't have anything wrong with him. My doctor says my blood pressure is way too high and the medicine isn't working very well because I have too much stress from taking care of Tom."

"I'm sorry to hear about your high blood pressure, and your doctor is correct by telling you that all of the

stress in your life is making that problem worse. I'm glad you're taking some steps now to find some options for helping yourself. I have a few more questions about your situation. Does Tom have any problems with walking or going up or down stairs, and does he drive?"

"No, he can walk just fine, and he still takes care of some little things around the house. Yes, he does still drive, and I know he probably shouldn't, but it's okay since it's just here around town. He just bought a new car, and he likes to drive it to visit friends or go to the store."

"Has Tom been told he has some type of dementia?"

"The doctor did tell him once early on that it might be, but when Tom heard that, he became terribly upset with the doctor. He told me on the way home from that visit that the doctor didn't know what he was talking about and if he ever mentioned it again, he wouldn't set foot in his office again, or let me go to him again, so I decided not to ever say anything about that again."

"I can certainly understand that. Please tell me some of the things that Tom does that are the most troublesome for you to handle now."

"Well, he's selling all my fur coats!"

"Do you know why he's doing that?"

"He says I won't need them anymore and that we have to prepare for dying since we're getting older. I just don't know what to say to him when he says and does things like this."

"Mrs. Samson, I think it would be a good idea for me to schedule a time to come to your home to assess just what your situation is and how to best interact with Tom. How would he react to my coming there to talk to both of you?"

"Well, you couldn't talk to him about dementia, because he would just get upset and probably throw you out of the house, but you could just come and pretend to be a friend of mine from the church who is interested in buying one of my fur coats. Then he'll be your best friend."

So that's what I did. I became a friend of Mrs. Samson's "from the church" who was interested in looking at the fur coats. Tom was indeed quite friendly and had the four coats spread out on the living room sofa for me to view. I dutifully tried them on and said I would have to think about it since it was such a big purchase.

"Well, you'll understand that I can't hold them for you unless you give me $100 down."

"Yes, I do understand that, and I appreciate the very low price you've put on these beautiful coats. May I ask why you're selling your wife's coats?"

"Why, it's because she won't need them anymore."

"Tom, it is getting to be the end of summer and cooler weather is coming soon. Are you moving south?"

"No, no, no. We're preparing for death. You know you've got to think ahead and we're not spring chickens anymore! I've got to make some hard decisions and start to get ready."

"So you don't think you'll still be around here this winter when your wife will need these coats?"

"Who knows? But she has plenty of other coats anyway, so it won't matter."

Tom went on to show me many other beautiful items in their home, and he could tell me the history of each one of them without missing a beat. His long-term memory was quite intact and he enjoyed talking about these things because it was so comfortable to him. He didn't have to struggle to find the memories because they were still there.

I eventually had the opportunity to sit and talk privately with Mrs. Samson and it was quite apparent she was under a great deal of the stress that is part of living with a spouse who has dementia and who is still quite high functioning.

When we talked about Tom's medications, she said that was another huge problem for her. On a daily basis Tom would take his medications out of the bottles and put them into a small bowl on the kitchen table. Then he would take them throughout the day when he sat down to eat. That method used to work for him, but as his dementia worsened, he would forget to take them, add more to the bowl the next day, and then she would have no idea what he had taken. He would not allow her to manage his medications, and this was also upsetting to her because she knew how important it was for him to be taking them regularly. When I asked her about the possibility of home nursing, she thought he might be willing to allow an agency nurse to come in and give him regular check-ups, as well as design a better method for taking his daily medications, but she had no idea of how to approach that subject with him. We decided to go on up to the kitchen where Tom was sitting eating a bowl of cereal, and see how far I could get with this idea. Tom had asked me when I first entered his home what it was I did for a living, and I had told him I was a nurse so I would now use that to talk to him about his medications.

"Boy, that's a nice big bowl of cereal you've got there, Tom!"

"I eat this much every single day." He did at one time, but now often skipped breakfast and was losing weight he could not afford to lose.

"Tom, do you recall that I said I was a nurse when I first came in here today?

"Yep, I sure do."

"Well, Tom, when your wife and I were talking just now, I was telling her we have this new program at church where nurses can help by going to people's homes to help them with whatever it is they need help with. We got to talking about her medicines, and she wants me to look through her medicines just to be sure everything is okay with them." Mrs. Samson handed me her shoebox of meds to inspect.

"Sounds like a nice thing to do. How much does it cost?" Tom continued to eat his cereal while we were talking.

"I'm not sure they have that all figured out yet, but I believe that if the person has insurance, then they could go ahead and bill for it, but if they don't have insurance, then there would be no charge. Would you like me to take a look at your medications also?"

"They're right here." He handed me his shoebox of meds, but didn't say anything about the twenty or so meds in the little bowl on the table in front of him.

"Tom, are these your meds here in this bowl, too?"

"Yep, those are the ones I'm taking today."

"Goodness! It looks like there are a few extra in here. How in the world can you tell them all apart?"

Tom tapped his temple with his finger. *"It's all right in here."*

"Tom, I'm a nurse, and I can't even tell what all these meds are! Take just this one little pill here. I see you have three of them in here: it's one of the pills for your heart, and I know that if you just happened to forget one afternoon that you already took it that morning and took another one, you could easily get very dizzy and fall. It's the same with your wife's medications, if she forgets she's already taken one of them, she could end up in the emergency room. You know what I think might be a better way for both of you? How about if one of those nurses comes here and brings one of those little medicine containers that has the days of the week listed on it? Then she could put all your medicines in the container and there wouldn't be any doubt about whether your wife forgot to take her meds?"

"Well, I guess that would be okay. I don't think we need it, but it's up to her." He gestured toward Mrs. Samson.

Another suggestion I gave to Mrs. Samson was to have home aides come in on a regular basis to help her with cleaning, as well as keep an eye on Tom and socialize with him in order to give her a break. These aides could do just a token amount of cleaning, and then spend an hour or so "off the clock" reminiscing with Tom about the very items he had had such a good time telling me about. That would allow her time to run errands or just get out of the house for awhile, as well as provide some help to Tom. Just being able to briefly step away from the stress and strain of wondering what Tom would do or say next could help reduce Mrs. Samson's blood pressure and allow her to return to him with renewed energy.

One of the most important suggestions I gave Mrs. Samson to help reduce some of her stress, was to stop arguing with Tom about things that really didn't matter. I suggested she pin a "sold" note to one fur coat at a time with a fake name and my phone number on it (in case he called to urge a speedy pick-up). Then, after a few days, hide the coat somewhere or put it in storage until she had "sold" all of them. I encouraged her to ask Tom's friends to step up and arrange for weekly outings for Tom that would give both of them a much needed break from each other.

We discussed Tom's driving which she reported as "still pretty good," but nonetheless worrisome. I suggested she have the doctor be the "bad guy" and ask him to order a driving test, not because of possible dementia, but "because some of the medicines he needed right now for his heart could impair his ability to drive *for* *awhile*." I stressed it was important to maintain Tom's sense of hope, control, and dignity as much as possible. Stopping the frequent arguments would help him feel more calm and in control. Using phrases such as "for awhile" would give him hope that it wasn't forever, and not constantly telling Tom that he was wrong, or that he had forgotten something, would maintain his dignity.

One of Mrs. Samson's biggest fears was that the doctor had told her he felt Tom should be placed in a facility now in order to reduce the stress on her. She obviously did not wish to do that despite her own failing health, and I felt Tom was still much too high functioning, too aware, to be placed in a facility this early in his dementia. I believed his reaction to being placed in a facility would be one of anger and probably result in physical aggression toward anyone attempting to make him stay there because he truly did not feel that he had any problems. Therefore, it would be crucial for both of them if she could change the ways she had been interacting with him so he would be more calm, which in turn would reduce her stress. I cautioned her, however, there is no way to predict how a person with dementia is going to act or react, and sometimes no matter what you do, it just doesn't work. For instance, she would not be able to prevent him from going up and down the basement stairs since their family room was downstairs and they used it daily.

Also, since Tom was still quite physically fit, he was at a high risk for walking or driving away and becoming lost. Aside from continually insisting on accompanying him, which she already knew wouldn't work with Tom, there was little else she could do aside from having the doctor order a driving test, possibly disabling the car, and making sure he had identification in his wallet at all times. Again, he was still too high functioning to agree to wear a wrist identification bracelet.

My heart ached for Mrs. Samson as we talked and the sheer enormity of her situation brought us both to tears as she struggled to find the strength to make the changes that would allow Tom to safely stay with her. Attempting to handle all of the issues arising with Tom by herself would certainly only serve to contribute to the decline of her own health, so it would be crucial for her to allow help from other sources as I had suggested.

My visit with Mrs. Samson was a very emotional one for me because of the many similarities I saw between her situation with Tom and my own mother's situation with my father. I have seen the sacrifices and the stresses forced upon my mother and I know how serious the threats are to her health. The challenges are many but they are not insurmountable, and I pray both of these women find the strength to overcome them.

"Do You Think We Should Still Take Our Vacation?"

Anna's husband, Alex, was asking for advice on whether he and Anna should take their yearly RV trip, or if they should stay home where things would be more familiar for Anna in the early stages of Alzheimer's. Anna kept asking him when they would be leaving but Alex was hesitant because he knew she would just forget about the trip later, and he wasn't sure if being in unfamiliar places would upset her.

I asked Alex to think about and answer several questions before deciding. First, what would be the potential benefits versus the potential risks of taking the trip? When you are living with a person with dementia, there are always safety risks regardless of whether they are at home or elsewhere. I told him if he felt they would both derive pleasure from the trip, and he was able to provide the constant vigilance that would be required with Anna, then they should try a short trip to test the waters. I advised him about some extra precautions that would need to be taken:

- Carry a cell phone at all times.

- Carry a current picture of Anna.

- Have both of them wear a MedicAlert bracelet (Anna's noting she has Alzheimer's and Alex's saying that he is the caregiver of a person with Alzheimer's).

- Have the name and the cell phone number sewn into all items of Anna's clothing.

- The RV would need to have some added locks to prevent Anna from wandering out at night, as well as keeping the doors locked while Alex was driving. It would be tragic if Anna forgot the RV was in motion and suddenly decided to go outside while Alex's attention was on his driving.

Some benefits of going on the trip would be that Anna would have increased stimulation and socialization that she wouldn't necessarily receive at home, but Alex would need to be able to recognize when Anna was becoming over-stimulated and needed to take a break from the journey. I felt that Alex could be building some wonderful memories for himself and the rest of his family, and he would feel good in knowing that he had helped to enrich Anna's life at that moment. Yes, she would eventually forget all about the trip, but every single, positive thing he did with Anna would have a benefit for her at that time. People with dementia begin to live in the moment, and the more wonderful moments you can give them, the happier they, and everyone around them are. If Alex felt Anna truly wanted to go on the trip, and he felt he was up for it as well, then I thought he could still create some wonderful travel memories.

Secondly, I advised Alex he would need to be aware of the warning signs of an illness and be prepared to take Anna to an emergency room for evaluation should the need arise. Some tips relative to that concern were:

- Keeping Anna hydrated and well rested would be key to helping her enjoy the trip.

- He would need to discuss the trip in advance with Anna's physician and have plans in place in case she required medication refills or copies of her medical records.

- It would be important for both of them to have their pertinent medical information as well as emergency contact information along with them, and easily accessible on the trip.

Third, Alex's travel plans would need to be very flexible. If he was constantly pushing to make it from point A to point B, then Anna would pick up on that stress and react in a like manner. If Anna clearly enjoyed stopping in one place for a few days, it would be nice if he were able to adjust the travel schedule to accommodate her. As with any person with dementia, the less you try to hurry them along, the happier you will both be.

If traveling in the RV was something they both had enjoyed in the past, the chances were good that they would still be able to experience many pleasurable moments. In the meantime, a short, two or three day trip would help Alex decide if both he and Anna were up for a much longer trip.

Safety In The Home

Safety is such a huge issue with any person with dementia and their family, as well as for the caregivers in facilities. In virtually every story in this book you will find issues that address different aspects of safety such as keeping the person with dementia safe from falls, from wandering, physical injuries, from dehydration or weight loss, or keeping the families and caregivers safe from physical harm by the person with dementia.

As I mentioned to Alex in the previous story, keeping Anna well-hydrated would be a key factor in how well she handled the trip. Increased confusion, lethargy, or even falls could indicate that Anna was dehydrated and she may not have a way to communicate that verbally to him.

Adults with intact brains probably don't spend much time thinking about hydration as they go about their daily activities, and I would guess that adults with dementia virtually never think about it, because they really cannot. That thirst mechanism in the brain that tells us when we're thirsty is often no longer functioning, or if it is, the person with dementia cannot figure out what to do about the signal. Yes, their mouth feels dry, but by the time they think of a glass of water, and make the effort to go get one, they often lose the thought along the way. Frequently handing them a glass of water, or favorite beverage just as if they had requested it, may encourage them to drink more often. Joining them with a glass for yourself is also often a good way to encourage them to drink.

"I'm going to have a glass of lemonade now, and I've brought one for you, too." Even if they say they're not thirsty, just putting the glass beside them and changing the subject can lead to them automatically just taking sips from it as they focus on something else. You can actually see a difference in how much more alert and awake they become when they are well-hydrated.

Some of the same problems surface with refusals to eat. They don't feel hungry so they may say they just ate breakfast/lunch/dinner. Again, the hunger mechanism isn't functioning properly or the brain isn't able to interpret the signal correctly. Avoid trying to re-orient them to the fact that they just got up so there is no way they could have eaten yet. Instead, say something like, *"Oh, I didn't realize that! Well, I'm going to sit down and eat something and I would love it if you would keep me company while I eat."* Then, change the subject, and after a short time and without asking any preferences, just place the food in front of them. If they say something like *"I told you I'm not hungry, I already ate!"* you can then say, *"I'm sorry! I guess I just automatically want to cook for two. Don't worry about it, just leave it there and I'll clear it away when I'm finished."*

As you sit down to enjoy your meal while engaging them in conversation, they may forget they're not hungry and simply begin to eat since the food is in front of them.

If weight loss is an issue, and it often is, then serving them their favorite foods can increase compliance greatly. If this person is on a special diet of some type, such as low cholesterol or low salt, then a balance must be found to allow them to enjoy their meals. It's much more difficult for families of a loved one with diabetes because compliance with their diabetic diet certainly isn't a high priority with that person who has dementia. They really could care less about such issues because they've forgotten why it's important. There are many good cookbooks out today that can give families tips on substitutions and on foods that can help control blood sugar. Of course, just keeping the home clear of any of the forbidden foods would be extremely helpful.

My father has been diagnosed with diabetes and although he does not require insulin yet, he has little regard for, or tolerance for efforts to reduce sweets and carbohydrates in his diet. Most of the time it has become such a challenge to persuade him to eat anything at all, that if he wants a favorite food that isn't good for his blood sugar, we give it to him. It becomes a question of quality of life versus quantity of life. Recently, Dad was telling me how he was looking forward to eating a piece of Mom's chocolate pie that she had just baked. He was getting as much enjoyment out of thinking about that pie as he would when he ate it later. I certainly wouldn't want to deprive him of that enjoyment even though I know it's not good for his blood sugar. Mom's challenge was to convince him to eat a large portion of his meal beforehand so that he wouldn't have room for such a huge piece of pie. At this stage, Dad still has many social graces intact so if everyone was sitting around the table enjoying the meal, then he would probably also eat well. These types of decisions are unique to every family's situation, and every family must be comfortable with the choices they make regarding diets.

An important part of safety is the issue of dignity. Care must always be taken to never treat this adult loved one like a child, even though what they are saying and how they are acting may be very childlike. I've heard of a term for that and it's called "infantilizing." When we reprimand or speak to an adult in a tone of voice reserved for children, then we are infantilizing that adult and they will always be aware of it whether they have dementia or not. Think for just a moment about the last time another adult treated you in a manner you perceived as being treated like a child. Did you appreciate it, or did you recognize it for what it was and resent it? Not only is it disrespectful, it is demeaning and counterproductive when you treat an adult with dementia like a child.

Doing child-like activities such as giving a woman with dementia a doll to carry is a completely different thing. If that woman believes the doll is a real baby and wishes to treat it as so, then you are not infantilizing her. If she knows it's a doll and you expect her, or encourage her to treat it like a real baby, then you are infantilizing her and she will likely become angry about it.

Let me tell you a story about how Bea reacted when she believed a staff person was treating her like a child. This story illustrates just how closely dignity is tied to the issue of safety.

"I'LL WHUP YOU!"

Bea was always such a little dynamo around the facility. When she was first admitted, she constantly wanted to be busy, so we would often give her "chores" to do such as pushing a non-electric floor broom down the hallways, or folding aprons or towels from the special basket of items we kept for residents to fold.

You will recall the story earlier when I told you about how Bea reacted to an employee attempting to vacuum a hallway where she had just run the non-electric floor broom. In Bea's mind, she certainly knew how to vacuum the floor, and she had done a good job, so this employee was clearly doing something wrong and needed to stop. If my employee had not stopped at Bea's request, then Bea would have interpreted that as a direct reflection on her capability to properly vacuum a floor, and she would have reacted in anger. In order to preserve Bea's dignity in that instance, the employee reacted appropriately by stopping her vacuuming and apologizing to Bea.

As most people with dementia are, Bea was quite astute at reading body language and interpreting the tone of voice used when speaking to her. She was standing just outside my office one day talking to an employee about doing some activity and I heard this employee respond to her in a patronizing voice: *"Now Bea, you know you can't do that anymore at your age."* I looked up in time to see Bea draw herself up to her full four foot height, glare up at the employee with her jaw locked, as she shook her finger beneath the employee's nose and said in a furious tone: *"Don't you talk to me that way. Just 'cause you're bigger than me doesn't mean I can't whup you when you need it!"* And as she stalked away, she smacked this employee on the behind to drive her point home. Bea recognized she was being treated like a child, and she didn't like it one bit.

I often use this story of Bea when training staff on dementia care because it illustrates so clearly how crucial it is for staff and families to be aware at all times of what their body language is saying, and what the tone of their voice conveys. Because of the brain damage, the person with dementia can no longer figure out what all the spoken words mean. Just as you and I do without even thinking about it, just as infants, and animals do, we all read body language. Body language and tone of voice speak louder to a person with dementia than the spoken words do, always, always, always!

Something else to consider on this topic is that when a person with dementia can no longer express their anger or frustration at someone with words (because their brain just can't find those words anymore) they will often resort to using their fists to get the point across. If Bea had lost the ability to say those words in anger, she would still feel the anger, and not being able to verbalize it would have resulted in her using her fists to make her point.

Driving With Dementia

In the early stages of dementia, driving can become a huge safety concern for families, and understandably so. Vision will be affected by dementia, with a gradual loss of peripheral vision and depth perception, and judgment is affected as well.

Asking an adult with dementia to hand over their independence and a portion of their pride by handing over their car keys is akin to lighting up a cigarette while standing next to an oxygen tank. You might get lucky and the tank will be fine, but you could also cause an explosion with serious injuries to anyone in the immediate vicinity; not to mention the fact that the person with dementia will likely forget they've handed over the keys and you may have to repeat the conversation multiple times unless you get creative with the excuses or the hiding of the keys.

My father doesn't drive very often any more, but if he wants to drive, there is very little likelihood that he will listen to anyone asking him to hand over the keys, and if he did hand them over without a fight, it would be a sign to us that he has "given up" and would be ready to check out of life completely. My family has learned they must beat him outside and physically sit in the driver's seat so he doesn't get the chance to get the keys in his hand. Once he has them in hand, he's much less likely to give them up.

Let me tell you the story of how I managed to convince a gentleman named Charles to willingly give me his car keys.

"Okay--You Can Have My Car Keys!"

Mary, a friend of mine who had a geriatric care management business was going out of town for two weeks and asked me to follow up on several of her clients while she was gone. She was especially concerned about Charles. She and Charles had been friends for many years, and now, following a surgical procedure, his dementia had progressed and he was still living alone, so he needed to be checked on frequently. She had recently been able to convince him to move to a lovely, upscale assisted-living facility near his home, but her biggest concern was that he was still driving. She told me she had not yet found a way to ask him for his car keys, and that if the opportunity presented itself to me, it would be a huge load off her mind if he were no longer driving. Charles didn't drive very often, and he never left town anymore, but the risk for injury is greatly compounded when dementia begins.

In briefing me about his situation, she warned me that Charles was an "outrageous flirt" and that he would likely hit on me when we met. I called the facility and made arrangements to come in to review his chart and also get staff input about their concerns with Charles. I then called Charles and he readily agreed to meet and talk to me at the facility when I told him Mary asked me to check in on him from time to time while she was out of town. I reminded him to mark the date and time on his calendar. *"It's a date!"* he said to me with great enthusiasm on the phone.

Charles' chart showed he was healing well from his recent surgery and the staff all enjoyed his sense of humor and easygoing manner. Their biggest concern was that he had left the facility twice in his car without telling anyone where he was going, and had not returned for several hours because he had gotten lost and couldn't find his way back. Once he returned to his old home where Mary found him, and the second time, a police officer noticed him driving too slowly and stopped him, and then escorted him back to the facility. They would all be relieved if he would surrender his car keys, so I planned to try to steer the conversation to that topic.

My first impression of Charles was that of a little rooster because he was a small man but walked with a little swagger with his chest puffed out. His full head of white hair was neatly combed and trimmed along with a small white mustache. He was in great physical shape despite his recent surgery, and I could see that he had taken pains to be well-groomed for our little meeting.

"Hello, Charles?"

"Yes, I'm Charles. And you must be Mary's friend. Mary didn't tell me I would be meeting such a beautiful woman, or I would have put my best duds on!"

"Yes, I'm Mary's friend, Cindy. Thank you, Charles. I'm happy to meet you. Mary has told me so many great stories about your long friendship. Why don't we sit down in this little library area and talk?"

"Beautiful lady, lead the way. I would follow you anywhere!"

"Charles, as you know, Mary has asked me to check in with you a few times while she's out of town. She wants to be sure you've recovered completely from your surgery. Tell me how you've been managing here."

Charles obliged by telling me about his physical limitations, and about the facility's food, rules, and regulations. To my relief, he said he was willing to remain there at least until Mary returned, but he wanted to go back home then. I decided at that point since he seemed so open and honest with me, to approach the driving issue.

"Charles, you're not able to drive yet are you?" I asked him this knowing that he's been told that he should not be driving by Mary and his surgeon.

"Well, technically, they say I shouldn't, but I don't have any problems with that at all. I feel just fine."

"Does that mean that you are driving?"

With a mischievous little grin he replied, *"Yes, I've been out a time or two. You won't tell on me now, will you?"*

"No, Charles, I won't tell on you, but if you continue driving, that really does put me in a difficult place."

"How so?" Since he is such a gentleman, he immediately became genuinely concerned when I said his actions were causing a problem for me.

"Well, as a nurse, I know that even while you feel fine, some of those medicines you need to take for awhile can cause sudden dizziness, because the anesthesia you had during your surgery takes a few months to work its way out of your system."

"So that's why the old eggs feel like they're scrambled sometimes!" He tapped his temple.

"Exactly! And Charles if you do drive during this recovery period, and you have an accident, even if it's not your fault, the nurses and doctors and Mary and I, everyone can be blamed for not helping you enough by reminding you to not drive or by not providing rides for you. Do you know that in any other situation, I would actually ask my patient to let me keep their car keys while they recover?"

"Now that's a scary thought."

"I agree! It is very scary to give up that little piece of independence, even for a short time. But you know, Charles, it's so much scarier for me to think about you driving while on those meds. I don't even want to think about what Mary would think of <u>me</u> if I couldn't keep you safe while she's gone."

"It's that serious, huh?"

"I'm afraid so."

"Well, hell. I can't let <u>you</u> get in trouble just because of me! Okay, you can have my car keys. That way you won't have to worry your pretty little head about anything with me!" He reached into his pocket and handed me his car keys.

"Charles, you are a true gentleman. Thank you for understanding my position and for caring about staying safe."

"You're welcome. Now what about if I need to go somewhere? Do I call you? Are you going to be my chauffeur?"

"They have a van service here, so you can first ask that woman at the desk area over there, and if it's somewhere out of town, then call Mary's number and I'll get the message and call you back. Here, I'll leave you a note with all that on it along with the phone number, okay?"

"Sounds like a plan, little lady. Now, when will I have the pleasure of talking with you again?"

Charles and I talked awhile about various topics and as I passed the nurses' station on my way out of the building, I stopped to let them know Charles had given me his car keys. We were all relieved and I gave myself a mental pat on the back for this very successful encounter. I could just imagine Mary's relief at hearing of that difficult task accomplished. The next afternoon, I received a phone call from the nurse at the facility saying: *"Cindy, just wanted you to know that Charles must have called the Chevy dealer this morning because they just delivered his new car!"*

The lesson learned? Don't expect anything to stay the way you left it when you're dealing with dementia!

Isolation

When you read the word "isolation" are you thinking I'm going to talk about the isolation of the person with dementia, or is your first thought that I am addressing the isolation that you, the caregiver, likely feel? Actually, it's both because there are few situations where they don't happen simultaneously. Let's talk first about your own social isolation.

Human beings were not meant to live isolated lives and when forced to do so, usually suffer in many ways. Please remember that you are not truly alone unless you choose to be, and I sincerely hope you choose to stay connected to other people outside of your home.

I completely understand how easy it is for a caregiver such as yourself to become isolated with your loved one. It just demands too much energy and effort to take them out of the house any more. With a probable struggle to get them bathed, dressed appropriately, into the car, and then to be constantly worried about when or if they will try to wander off, say or do inappropriate things, or become upset, it's just much easier to keep them at home where things are more familiar to them and they aren't upset as easily. I don't blame you. I would feel the same way, and why choose possible chaos when you could avoid it? I would ask, however, that you consider the possible negative impacts of social isolation on yourself and your loved one now, and plan for ways you might reduce the chances of it happening to you.

The reality of social isolation is that not only do the caregivers and the lives of every family member become more and more isolated, they suffer higher rates of depression and illness. It's not at all unusual for the caregiver of a person with dementia to die first and the reason is because of the increased stress. Caregivers must make a conscious effort and commitment to take care of themselves and to make it a priority and a habit. If they don't, the disease that is dementia slowly dissolves their life just as surely as it is dissolving the brain of their loved one.

Social isolation of caregivers usually happens over time and is unintentional, and I have a pretty good idea as to why it happens. Do you remember seeing how horses pulling carriages must have those "blinders" on so they can't use their peripheral vision? They are forced to focus only on the road ahead and not look at what is beside them that could help them or harm them. This is what often happens to you caregivers who are living with loved ones with dementia; you have put on your own special pair of "blinders" in order to just get through the next hour or the next day safely with this person. And in doing so you've become isolated from friends, families, activities you once enjoyed, and social outlets such as church or outings with friends.

Stop and think for a moment. Have you put "blinders" on? Is your daily course so focused that you cannot stop to enjoy your friends or activities along the way? If so, I urge you to think of ways to allow yourself some freedom from those self-imposed "blinders."

Step back and take an honest look at your life and then ask some trusted friends or relatives for their opinion as to whether or not you are becoming more and more isolated, more focused on your loved one, or more depressed. If they tell you what you don't want to hear, I beg of you to listen, and then begin to take the steps necessary to give yourself back some of your life.

Think about this: If you were on an airplane with this loved one, and the cabin pressure suddenly decreased so the oxygen bags dropped down, whose oxygen mask would you put on first? Your own or your loved one's? You know I'm going to tell you the correct answer is to put your own mask on first, just as you know the reason why that's so. You are no help to anyone when you sacrifice your health, your self, your sanity, or your joy for the sake of another person. And guess what? Your loved one will suffer right along beside you because you are not able to be the best caregiver to them when you are suffering in any way. Why should you both suffer more when you can make a conscious decision to relieve some of that suffering by keeping yourself mentally, physically, and spiritually healthier?

Let's examine some ways you might accomplish that for yourself. Does your loved one sleep for extended periods of time? If so, rather than trying to force them up at a time when they *used to* arise, use that time to do the things you find difficult to do when they are up and about:

- Call your friends for a chat on the phone while enjoying a cup of coffee. Or, ask one of your friends to come to your home on a regular basis to spend time with you while your loved one is not requiring your attention.

- Enjoy some quiet time to read or work on a project.

- Get all the housework done so you won't have to worry about it later.

- Use the quiet time to catch up on paying bills or organizing financial affairs.

- If you value attending church but have been unable to, ask your clergy to visit you in your home. And please don't discount another type of "counseling" for yourself: psychological counseling. Again, numerous studies have shown huge benefits for caregivers who utilize this resource to reduce their many burdens.

- Sleep in late! If you are sleep-deprived, you will need to add more sleep-time with naps or by sleeping late. Many, many studies show that a simple, chronic lack of sleep negatively affects every aspect of your life. Taking a nap later in the day when your loved one is resting is also a great idea. As long as your loved one isn't up all night and sleeping all day, allowing them to sleep longer will help both of you feel better.

- Allow friends, family, or a local Meals On Wheels program to bring you meals on a regular basis. The time and effort that saves you will contribute greatly to your own comfort.

It will also contribute to your well-being to give yourself some much needed time away from your loved one; to actually get out of the house and do something you enjoy. As mentioned above, this might be accomplished by putting together a network of friends of your loved one to come to visit on a regular basis, every day or every other day. This can be one of the best ways to keep them socialized, as well as giving you some free time.

In order for these visits to be successful however, there are some ground rules everyone needs to know. These should not be lengthy visits (even if they are 20-30 minutes in length), they would serve to prevent that isolation, as well as give you a short break.

Choosing the best time of day is important. For instance, does your loved one seem more calm and alert before lunch or after? Choose the best option there, and try to adhere to it.

What types of interactions did this friend have with your loved one? If it was only to get together to play golf, obviously there will come a time when that's no longer possible. If that's the case now, how about if this golfer friend simply brings his golfing equipment and they discuss ways to correct a defective swing, or talk about if the new golf balls really do drive farther? Asking the person with dementia for their opinion on something they used to know a lot about will help them feel normal again, and that's always a good thing.

Bringing out a photo album or other memorabilia is a great way to reminisce with this loved one. People must take care never to point to a picture or item and ask the person with dementia, "Do you remember...?" If the person with dementia cannot remember, it frustrates them, and that's exactly the opposite reaction you want. Always, always, always give this person clues as you converse with them such as the following examples:

A. *"Stanley, your old golfing buddy, Marv, is here to see you for just a short visit..."* Now Stanley doesn't have to try and then fail to come up with Marv's name as well as the hobby they shared, and since you said it was a "short" visit, he won't be stressed to think he has to entertain Marv for a long period of time.

B. *"Oh Mom, look at this picture. I remember when Dad took this picture of me and my dog, Scruffy. I look like I'm about seven years old here."* If she doesn't seem to recall anything about the picture, simply move on to the next one. Don't try to force a memory because it will only frustrate her.

C. *"Oh for heaven's sake! You and I look like we've had too much to drink in this picture taken down at the shore!"* If they say that isn't the two of you, that it's someone else, simply go along with them and move on: *"Oh, you're probably right, now that you mention it, I think it's..."*

D. *"What do you think about this new fishing fly I tied? Do you think I'll catch the biggest trout with it? We'll have to set a date to get down to the stream to test it out."* It really doesn't matter at this point that you'll never go fishing with him again (he doesn't know that), what matters at this moment is that you've asked his opinion, and that you want to go fishing with him, something he loves to do. You have just helped him remember this hobby and how much he enjoys it and your companionship and you have just made him happy.

E. *"I remember that time when your car broke down, Stan, and you and I had to walk three miles in that rainstorm. I still liked that old Chevy though."* Now you can spend the next few minutes discussing cars if that's a subject he loves to talk about. Stan will probably tell you things he's said over and over again the last few times you visited, but it's essential that you act as if this is the first time you've heard them. Your goal is to have a good visit with Stan, to have him enjoy your company, and to entertain him. All of those things will happen if Stan believes he's having a normal, new conversation with you. Nobody likes to be told they're repeating a story.

If the dementia has advanced to a point where the person is not able to converse about what they remember, then finding what appeals to the senses is what will bring them happiness and comfort. It can simply be a picture, or a soft, stuffed animal. Watching fish swim in an aquarium often contributes to a sense of calm, as does listening to some favorite music. Also, don't ever underestimate just how powerful it can be to simply hold someone's hand as you sit quietly beside them. Any time you stimulate their brain by introducing a different topic or sensation, you are preventing the isolation that keeps them locked into their own confused minds.

Some other ways to help keep your loved one socialized:

•Ask family members to schedule regular visits, as well as assist you on an occasional doctor visit or shopping trip with your loved one. This also helps those family members see some of the challenges you are faced with daily. Tell them it's payback for all those dirty diapers you had to change for them!

•Give adult daycare a few tries before discounting it. Nearly every family I have counseled has told me, "Oh no, (s)he would never stay there even for an hour." When they actually tried it, and worked through the adjustment period with the staff, they were very glad they had and it usually always worked out well. This is one of the most important decisions you can make for the well-being of both of you.

By choosing to spend time reading this book, you've already demonstrated that you can and did make a good decision to help yourself and your loved one. Please continue on along this pathway to find what works best for you and your unique situation. But please don't give up. What doesn't work this week, may work out well next week.

The Mack Truck Heading Straight Toward You--Fearing For Your Own Safety

In my varied nursing career, I have known and loved many, many people with dementia. Conversely, I've also known and feared a few people with dementia. Fear can be a good thing when it warns you to make some changes you don't really want to, but which, in the end, will protect you and your loved one from unintentional harm.

This client family was having a great deal of difficulty dealing with the father/husband, Bryce, who had suffered a series of strokes in the frontal lobe of his brain that led the doctors to diagnose "frontal lobe dementia." He was still able to function independently a great deal of the time and didn't have much short-term memory loss, but he was now displaying more and more frequent episodes of agitation and aggression toward them. His team of physicians was working hard to reduce the aggression with medication, and the family needed to hear some suggestions from me as to what they could do to reduce or prevent the frightening outbursts.

Stella, the daughter, had called me because her father was becoming increasingly angry and accusatory toward her mother. She related that he had chased her mother out of the house, yelling at her, and when her mother had called Stella at her home nearby to come and help calm him down, her father had begun yelling at her and had physically attacked her. Naturally this was quite devastating for Stella and she reported tearfully that *"he never showed any remorse or seemed to be sorry for it at all."* It was my unpleasant duty to inform this family that when the frontal lobe of the brain is damaged, unpredictable, aggressive, and dangerous behaviors can become common. I told them they could no longer count on their father/husband having the ability to feel remorse for anything he did, and that the most important thing to consider now was their own continued safety.

Antipsychotic, anti-anxiety, and anti-depressant drugs can help take the edge off those behaviors, but it's always a guessing game as to how the person will respond to those medications, or for how long they will be effective. Then again, what works well for this month, may not work at all next month as the dementia progresses. It's essential to have a physician willing to work with you on this huge safety issue.

A factor complicating Bryce's treatment was that he was continuing to drink alcohol with his medications, despite being told by the physicians that it would be dangerous to do so. He was still physically and mentally able to supply himself with alcohol, and he repeatedly denied his alcohol consumption to his physicians. Even when they were successful in temporarily getting rid of all the alcohol in the house, he would search through medicine cabinets to drink any liquids he found there.

This family needed to have a safety plan in place for all members of the family. The women were not to be left alone in the house or car with him because they could never be sure when he might suddenly decide they had done something against him and become aggressive toward them. Since there were two adult sons who lived in the home with him, that could be accomplished relatively easily.

It was also extremely important for all members of the family to stop arguing with Bryce or trying to re-orient him when he insisted he was right. He no longer had the ability to understand reason, and every time they argued with him, they would risk triggering his aggression.

This family also needed to decide who they could trust to talk privately with Bryce to get him to sign a durable healthcare power of attorney as well as a legal power of attorney for his finances. They felt certain he no longer trusted any of them, but that he might still trust his attorney, so plans were made to accomplish those extremely important tasks. Bryce had already, with the reduced impulse control common in frontal lobe damage, gone out and purchased a new $40,000 truck. He had also called several contractors to redo a beautiful new patio, and had even talked about purchasing a local restaurant/hotel when he found it was for sale. It was imperative that someone besides Bryce have the ability to control the money, as well as have the ability to make healthcare decisions when needed for him.

Thankfully, Bryce did not argue about who would drive when they went anywhere in the car, and when they were not driving, the car keys always seemed to magically get lost at home.

I asked the family if Bryce had any hobbies or interests, and the only things they could come up with were that he was very fond of the cat, and he would water the houseplants numerous times a day. He had been a hard worker his entire life and had never taken time to develop hobbies, and his interest in sports on television was waning.

Stella recounted how he had been so impressed with her large, flat-screen television that the family had purchased one slightly smaller for him for Christmas. Instead of displaying happiness in receiving the expensive gift, Bryce had bitterly complained about how small it was, even though it was twice as large as his current television screen. They were berating themselves for not getting the larger one in the first place and were considering "upgrading" the television. I suggested they just not go there with the guilt. I told them there was an equal chance that had they given him the larger one, he may have bitterly complained about them spending so much money on something so large. "Should'a-would'a-could'a" won't serve any purpose whatsoever in the day-to-day caring for a person with dementia. It only increases the guilt the caregivers are feeling. Families so often find themselves continually running around after these people just to do damage control, that there is little time to know in advance what would be best. That's not to say that families should not plan for emergencies in advance, but stressing over the water that has already gone under the bridge in the form of unpredictable behaviors won't serve any useful purpose whatsoever. Just don't go there.

In this family's situation, the possibility of bringing a second cat into the house was discussed, as well as adding more plants for Bryce to water. Bryce's wife expressed irritation at the fact that he kept watering a large artificial plant, and she had even once reminded him it was artificial (which resulted in an angry confrontation) so she now knew well enough to stay quiet about it and let him water it. She would also now go around and empty the excess water from the drip pans instead of berate him for watering them too often. She was learning the difficult lesson of how and when to pick the battles. Allowing him to do things that seemed to comfort or calm him would help keep him in a good frame of mind, which in turn would help everyone around him relax.

Because he had no hobbies, Bryce's family would be continually challenged to find enjoyable things to occupy his time and his mind. Putting the photograph albums out on the coffee table would allow family members more opportunities to reminisce about good times with him, which would help reduce his agitation.

I also urged this family to begin checking out nearby dementia facilities and when they found one they felt comfortable with, they should put Bryce's name on the waiting list. There would be no way to predict when a medical crisis would occur which would necessitate a sudden move to such a facility, and being prepared in advance would save them a lot of trauma and worry. Of course, there would be no way to predict which type of facility would be appropriate for Bryce at the time of the medical crisis, but having done the initial paperwork, they would be far ahead of the game if and when it became necessary.

If Bryce were mobile at the time of admission, then a secure or locked facility would be needed since he would likely try to go home many times. If he were not mobile but required skilled nursing care, then a nursing home or skilled nursing facility would be required.

I stressed to the family they should never hesitate to call on the local police to intervene when and if Bryce was putting their lives, or his own life, in danger. If that happened, then there was a chance Bryce could be transported to the local hospital's psychiatric unit and admitted involuntarily for a short period of time. As traumatic as that would be for everyone involved, it would be less traumatic than the injury or death of one of them at Bryce's hands.

I told this family that in many ways this would be the toughest stage for them to go through with Bryce. At some level he knew he was having memory problems and he was scared, which he then likely displayed as frustration or anger. He really could not help himself when he did those impulsive things that got everyone around him stirred up and angry. He was still an adult who could make decisions such as whether to drink or not, so legally, there was little they could do about it unless they had him declared incompetent. He was still quite mobile so the threat of him wandering away and getting lost was a daily concern, and there were times when he refused to even carry a wallet when he went out. As his dementia progressed, he would lose the ability to do some of these things, and the family would then be faced with a new set of problems to solve, but for now, keeping themselves and Bryce safe was a primary concern.

Equally important was the need for Bryce to maintain some degree of control over his environment, and to be treated with dignity and respect by others. Any time he suspected he was being completely controlled or treated with anything less than respect and dignity, he was sure to react with agitation and aggression. Bryce's family would need to seek that delicate, ever-shifting balance between Bryce's safety, dignity, and volatile temper and their own safety and ability to live with his challenging behaviors. At some point, facility placement would become the best option if only to keep them all safe from the dementia that was destroying Bryce's ability to control his temper and his actions. They would need to be strong enough, and love Bryce enough, to implement that decision.

If the situation you're living in with a loved one with dementia is causing you to experience fear, please take that as a sign to take control and make the moves necessary to help keep you and that loved one safer. Oftentimes that means admitting your loved one to a facility even though you may have promised each other to never take that step. Life has a way of changing the plans and the rules in the middle of the game, so please don't beat yourself up over a decision that you found the courage to make.

Just as an oncoming truck unexpectedly swerving straight toward you for a head-on collision would cause you great harm and possibly death if you didn't make a decision to change your course, there is no way you can predict how the dementia will change your loved one's brain, and thereby change the rules of your lives. If the warning signs are there, and the behaviors of your loved one have caused you fear, please don't let your loved one become that truck; make the decision to stay safe, and move forward on an altered course.

"I'm Going To Kill You!"

This is another story about safety issues, but it's also a story about enduring love.

Robert would bring his wife, Anna, to our medical practice for her ongoing care and treatment. Anna was in the later stages of dementia, but Robert was determined to take care of her at home, and it was touching to see just how gentle and compassionate he was with her.

Robert owned a store in a neighboring town, and he would get Anna up and dressed every morning, then bring her to the store with him while he worked. He had a cot set up in the back room of the store for when she got tired and needed to nap, and he kept all of her favorite foods on hand and encouraged her constantly to "have just a bite, sweetie."

Robert's gentle sense of humor was an essential part of his caregiving skills. It was typical of him to always see the humor in everything and I recall one day when he brought Anna in to the office. When he removed his coat I could see big splotches on his shirt where something had faded the color in places. He noticed my glance and with a grin said: *"I discovered this is the result I get if I pour the laundry softener on the clothes instead of waiting for the water!"*

One day as I was preparing to take her blood pressure in the office, Anna, who usually didn't speak much at all, turned to Robert and in a growly, menacing, monotone voice said: *"I'm going to kill you. I'm going to get a knife and I'm going to kill you."*

Robert's calm response was: *"Yes dear, I understand. When we get home you can think about that then."*

I asked him if she threatened him often like this, and he said: *"Only once in awhile, but when we get home she forgets about it. I'm very thankful for that!"*

I doubt if Anna would have had the physical strength to do much damage to Robert even if she happened to get hold of a knife, but when the person with dementia is a man, he presents a much bigger danger to everyone around him.

I feel Robert was doing an amazing job of nurturing Anna as he cared for her and at the same time, he was using his wonderful sense of humor to reduce his own emotional stress.

"How Can We Convince Mom To Move Here?"

RuthAnn was calling me to ask this question because she and her sister Marie, who lived on the West coast, had decided the safest thing for their mother with early dementia was to move her to an assisted-living facility near RuthAnn. Their mother was currently living in a retirement village in her own trailer in another state where she had resided for many years. She had lots of neighbors who checked on her regularly, but she had refused in-home help when RuthAnn had tried to arrange it. The neighbors had "rescued" her mother several times when she had fallen while outside, and had voiced their concerns about her safety on numerous occasions. The daughters were concerned about how to get their mother moved in the most effective and compassionate way since it was clear she could no longer live on her own so far away.

Their mother had admitted that her memory wasn't as good as it used to be, but had already told them she did not wish to move anywhere. In a telephone conference call, I offered options to these two loving and concerned daughters about how to accomplish the daunting tasks involved in getting their mother to agree to move, and then in planning the actual move.

RuthAnn was planning to fly down to visit her mother the following week and I suggested during her visit she finalize plans for the durable healthcare power of attorney, and then make sure she accompanied her mother to her doctor's appointment. She would need to sign a form for release of her mother's records, and if she had decided on which facility to move her mother into, to have the records forwarded there. She could do these tasks without ever mentioning the move to her mother.

To ease into the subject of the move, RuthAnn needed to make many "I" comments to her mother such as: *"I would love it if you could come for a visit. It's been so long and the grand-children really miss you."*

She should avoid any arguments, try to remain calm, and always present a relaxed, smiling presence with lots of hugs. She could wait for openings in the conversation and interject comments such as: *"I would love to cook for you..." or "I remember what a nice time we had shopping at that big mall near me the last time you visited."*

These kinds of statements would help remind her mother how nice it would be to be closer to her daughter, and to enjoy the rest of the family again without putting pressure on her to make a decision.

While there, RuthAnn could also make arrangements with a real estate agent to prepare for the final move a month or so in advance, again, without upsetting her mother by telling her in advance.

To help keep her mother safer in the interim, I suggested she arrange for some in-home care in the form of a "cleaning lady" since her mother was now using a walker to get around. She could give this to her mother as a "gift" and could be present when the person came the first few times. This would help her mother get used to another person coming into her home, and by the time RuthAnn left, she would hopefully be comfortable with this arrangement and allow it to continue. It would give the daughters a bit more peace of mind knowing there would be another person there to check on their mother as they finalized the moving plans.

RuthAnn returned two weeks later and reported her visit went very well. She was able to maintain a calm and loving demeanor and her mother had admitted it would be nice to be closer to the family. When RuthAnn had said she knew of a really nice place her mother could live (while keeping the house she currently had just in case she didn't like it) her mother had agreed that "might be a good idea." The "cleaning lady" was in place and RuthAnn and Marie made plans for the final move to take place in approximately one month. They would both fly there for the packing up, then Marie would drive her mother back, while RuthAnn would fly back and place her mother's personal items in the facility in advance of her arrival.

In the interim, they would both, along with other family members, call regularly to express their joy at her "decision" to move "even if it's only temporary" because they missed her so much. At the same time, they could tell her of all the wonderful things they could do together once she arrived. If she was having a "bad day" where she had completely forgotten the plan to move, they weren't to remind her of it, but to simply apologize, say they must have gotten it wrong, and go on to a safer subject such as: *"Oh, I'm sorry I misunderstood, I guess I thought you were moving here when you're just going to be visiting. I'm just so happy to be seeing you again. I have so many great things to talk to you about!"*

RuthAnn reported that things went well with the caregiver for a couple of weeks until one day she got a call from her mother whom she described as being "on the warpath." She was furious that the caregiver was there, that she just wanted to be left alone, and threatened to move away and not tell anyone where she had gone. As I had discussed the possibility of this scenario happening previously with RuthAnn, she had instructed the caregiver to leave, but to return the following morning as if nothing had happened. Fortunately, her mother was scheduled to see her doctor the next day for one final time before the move, so I asked RuthAnn to instruct the doctor's office to have her mother tested for a urinary tract infection. If the tests were positive, an antibiotic could be started quickly and her mood and behaviors would return to baseline. The difficulty would be for her to actually remember to take a new pill on a daily basis. It turned out that her mother did have a urinary tract infection and she was successfully treated with an antibiotic. To everyone's relief, she had forgotten her outburst against the caregiver and did allow her back into her home the next day.

RuthAnn and Marie reported that the big move was successful, but stressful for their mother, as expected. They had chosen a small assisted-living facility near RuthAnn since it seemed more "home-like," and there was a family member with her almost constantly for the first several days while she adjusted. The family members all made a huge fuss over her and continually told her how wonderful it was that she had decided to move there, so this made the transition much easier for her to make. These daughters had managed to accomplish their goal of moving their mother across country in a safe, loving, and dignified manner. By learning and utilizing these new ways of interacting with their mother, it all soon became second nature to them:

- Instead of trying to continually re-orient her, getting into her reality, agreeing with her, and then changing the subject.

- Making numerous "I" statements to convey to their mother just how wonderful she made them feel.

- Praising their mother at every opportunity for all of the right things she was doing, and the right decisions she had made.

- Giving their mother lots of physical affection in the form of hugs and smiles.

- Allowing their mother to have hope that if she didn't like the new arrangements, she could go back. Although delay tactics would be used if their mother decided to go back.

- Keeping their body language calm, relaxed, and open when they interacted with her in any way.

RuthAnn and Marie's mother settled in at the assisted-living facility and soon forgot about her "home" so far away. As happens with most people with dementia who are placed into facilities, eventually the facility becomes home to them and the requests to "go home" become fewer and fewer.

"When Will I Have To Make The Nursing Home Decision And What Do I Need To Look For In A Facility?"

These are questions I am frequently asked by clients as they struggle to care for their loved ones at home. Spouses may have promised to "never" place each other in a nursing home, only to find that because of their own failing health and the highly physical burden of caring for a person with dementia, they now have no other choice. The guilt they feel is crushing and relentless. They are not only watching their loved one's condition deteriorate, but they can't help but question if they had just kept them at home for another month or so, would they have been able to prevent this or that negative occurrence from happening.

In as gentle a way as I can, I try to help these families find some answers. There is no perfect answer for every family situation and there is no way to tell how "right" that decision will be once it is made.

In the story you just read about RuthAnn's mother, the decision to place her in a facility was not the most difficult decision for that family. The daughters both knew they could not safely care for her in their homes, and the bigger question for them was _when_ to place her, and how to accomplish it in a way their mother could believe it was actually her own decision to move.

"How will I know when it's time?" This is another question I am frequently asked, usually by a spouse caregiver who already has, for various reasons, decided that placement in a facility is necessary. They just want to delay it as long as possible and need some sign that the time has arrived. That sign will be different for everyone. For some people "the straw that breaks the camel's back" will be their loved one's loss of ability to maintain urine or fecal continence. In fact, incontinence is one of the leading reasons for admission to facilities. This embarrassing task is often complicated by factors such as the physical frailty of the caregiver; they're just not able to do all the bending, lifting, or twisting required in removing and replacing lower body garments and underwear. It's further complicated if the person with dementia is being resistant or wants to do it themselves. Women are usually better at the "mechanics" of this type of task simply because they've changed and cleaned the bottoms of their children countless times and know how it's to be done. But, cleaning the bottom of an adult who may be embarrassed, resistant, possibly combative, or all of the above, is quite another matter.

Sometimes incontinence problems are complicated simply by not knowing the mechanics. I recall a gentleman who told me he was quite willing and able to help keep his wife at home despite her increasing incontinence, but after she developed three urinary tract infections in a row, he learned for the first time that he needed to be wiping her peri-area from front to back. He was unknowingly contributing to her acquiring the urinary tract infections simply by not knowing that women need to be wiped and cleaned from front to back to avoid bringing bacteria from the rectal area forward to the urethral area.

When the family caregiver is a son or daughter, the mere thought of tending to a parent in such an intimate task can be overwhelming, and they are unable to do it. Personally, I would have difficulty helping my father change his urinary catheter when the time comes that he can no longer do that for himself. I might be able to overcome my embarrassment and find a way to help him overcome his embarrassment, but that's a place I hope to never go, because that's my dad, that's not some patient I've helped with those tasks many times in my nursing career.

It's often easier for people to accept having a stranger such as a nurse or an aide help them with personal hygiene than it is for a son or daughter, however, there are many, many family members out there who are willing and able to perform these tasks. Many times the determination of who performs those tasks is made by the ability, or inability, to pay for those services.

I ask families to focus on what they can do instead of what they cannot do for their loved one. If they cannot bring themselves to bathe, dress, or change the briefs of their loved ones, then don't beat themselves up over it. Make the decision that is needed to accomplish those tasks whether it is to hire daily aides, or to admit their loved one to a facility. They will then have the freedom to help enrich the life of their loved one in a multitude of other ways, as a son, daughter, or spouse instead of as a full-time caregiver.

Even though it may feel like it, it's truly not the end of the world to have to admit a loved one to a facility. I have seen many people with dementia actually improve after admission to a facility, but it also depends greatly upon the facility. Some things to consider when searching for the best facility for your loved one with dementia include:

- Is there a separate, secure dementia unit? This is essential if your loved one is still mobile and able to "escape."

- Just as important, the facility needs to have staff who have on-going dementia training, and who you observe interacting in a happy and positive way with all residents. The presence of staff that has been trained in how to successfully redirect someone's attention from wanting to go home to something else, will determine how content those loved ones are in the facility. Acknowledging their discomfort, showing empathy, and then redirecting the conversation, or simply giving the person with dementia some hope that they will be able to go home can calm and comfort them.

- The activities department at the facility should have different levels of activities posted for dementia residents who may all be in different stages of their dementia.

- What is the physical layout of the facility? Would it be easy for a person with dementia to navigate? The unit should be constructed in such a way that it allows people to walk unimpeded for exercise. I once did a staff training in a large nursing home that had two separate dementia units. One was for higher- functioning mobile residents, and the other was for those residents whose dementia had progressed to the point where they were no longer able to walk without assistance. What made it especially nice was that the higher- functioning dementia residents didn't have to continually navigate around wheelchairs and geri-chairs, and the unit was quite calm, stress free, and clutter free. In the non-mobile unit, the presence of wheelchairs, geri-chairs, laundry carts, and such didn't impede the mobility of those residents, or distress them. Their worlds had shrunken to the immediate space around them and they were being tended to by staff trained to provide stimulating activities geared to those levels of interaction.

- Does the facility have one or more physicians who come to the facility on a regular basis to see their patients? It's fine if the families wish to continue driving their loved one to see the primary care physician, but there will come a time when that can no longer be done safely due to declining abilities and the mental trauma it can cause to a person with dementia. So, it's much easier on everyone if the physicians come into the facilities to see the patients.

The difficult nursing home decision will always be affected by any number of factors for each family. Focus on moving forward and believing you have made the right decision by realizing what positive results can be seen from that decision:

- You can now become the wife, husband, son, daughter, sister, or brother once again instead of having to focus on every physical aspect of your loved one's care.

- You will now have the extra time to devote to having quality visits where you are arriving refreshed and rested. This helps ensure you are able to maintain your calm, relaxed demeanor while you visit. Never forget that your calm and serene demeanor benefits your loved one immeasurably.

- Your loved one is receiving round-the-clock care and social stimulation on a much higher level than could be provided at home. Simply observing the constantly changing scenes before them is a type of stimulation that can benefit them.

- You are still an advocate for your loved one and can be as involved in the day-to-day care as you wish to be, and as the facility allows.

- You can find some semblance of order and normalcy to your daily routine when you aren't forced to be acutely aware of what your loved is doing from minute to minute.

While the facility placement decision will usually be a difficult one no matter what the underlying reasons are, if the family can focus on what good things can come of it, the transition will be easier on everyone involved. As I mentioned previously, I have seen many residents improve dramatically (physically and mentally) when admitted to a facility. If you are able to focus on the improved relationship you can now have with your loved one, you will be able to accept your difficult decision a little more easily.

Let's Talk About Falls

Many times the nursing home placement decision is made due to a crisis such as a fall that results in injuries to the person with dementia. Please, please, please know that *every* person with dementia will fall eventually as their dementia progresses. The messages from the brain to the legs and feet will be short-circuited and what begins as an occasional stumbling will progress to falls. You will never be able to predict when that might happen, but being aware of what is coming, there are steps you can take to help keep your loved one safer from falls in your home. Again, please notice that I have used the word "safer" and not the word "safe." Know that falls will occur and your goal will be to minimize the number of falls, and the injuries that might occur. There are a number of things you can do in your home to reach this goal:

- Remove all throw rugs. Walk through your home in a shuffling manner and see just how easily your feet will catch every rug you encounter.

- Keep all clutter cleared off the floors. This includes stacks of magazines, bags or boxes of items, clothing, or shoes on the floor.

- Block access to all stairs. With the vision changes that occur, they are unable to see stair steps and will fall up or down them.

- Be aware of the condition of the shoes they are wearing. Are the heels worn to one side or are the laces too long? Do the shoes still fit or are they now too big and flop on their feet as they walk? Loss of weight will cause foot size to shrink.

- If they use a walker or a cane, check the tips of those to be sure they're not catching in the carpet.

- If this person has lost weight, their clothing will be too big and could fall down as they walk. Even if you use a belt or suspenders, it's not comfortable to wear clothing that is too big, and just being distracted by this feeling could lead to a fall.

- Place favorite items within easy reach for this loved one. Even if they can still reach up to that second shelf to get the cereal bowl, just that little extra stretch could put them off balance enough to fall.

- Get rid of glass-topped furniture. If they happen to fall onto a coffee table, the injuries will be less severe if glass is not involved.

- Consider what might be done to prevent a beloved, elderly pet from causing a fall. If the cat or dog likes to lay in the sunshine on the floor, but presents a trip hazard because they won't move if someone steps near them, then remove the reason for them to be there. Close the drapes, or place a comfortable "bed" for them somewhere your loved one won't be walking.

- Dizziness may become a factor. Has your loved one been checked for orthostatic hypotension? This is where the blood pressure drops quickly when they move from a sitting to standing position, or rising from the bed to stand up. They can't necessarily tell you they feel dizzy, but they will fall if they try to walk while dizzy.

- If this loved one has become fatigued, they are at a much higher risk of falling as they walk. If you feel they are becoming tired, try to encourage them to sit and rest by giving them a photo album or turning on the TV for a favorite show. Better yet, you sit down with them and rest!

- Dehydration is always a huge concern. Even if they are slightly dehydrated, it will affect their ability to walk properly. I discuss this in detail elsewhere in the book.

- Many medications can cause slight dizziness, so you must be watchful when any new medication has been started. Sometimes the dizziness is mild and temporary, but it can still contribute to a fall.

"I Don't Want To Stay Here!"

When a person with dementia has been isolated at home with just a few familiar faces around them on a daily basis, admission to the very social atmosphere in a facility can initially increase their confusion as well as their anxiety. But, often within a few weeks, the facility becomes the most familiar place to them, and it becomes "home" to them. Consistent kindness, patience, and redirection by a well-trained staff will help the person with dementia become more willing to relax and maintain their hope they will return "home."

One newly-admitted woman in our facility would come to my office several times a day and ask me to please call her daughter to come to take her home. Knowing that she held her doctor in high esteem, and that her social graces were still intact, here is how I would respond to her (always with a big smile on my face and in my voice): *"Hi Maria! You're looking lovely today! Did you say you wanted me to call your daughter?"*

"Thank you. Yes, I need to call my daughter, Anna, to tell her to come here and pick me up and take me home. I certainly can't stay here!"

"Oh, Maria! You know, I was just checking a few minutes ago, and we still don't have your lab results back. I spoke with your doctor about that and he's pretty adamant about the fact that he doesn't want you

to leave here until he's sure you're in the best shape possible! He said it might take another day or so until we get them all back, and then he'll release you to go home."

"Oh, but I don't want to stay here!"

"Oh, I know you don't want to stay here, Maria, and I'm so sorry about that. But you know what a good doctor he is, and how he cares about you. Besides, your doctor and Anna have picked this beautiful place for you to wait. It's not a nursing home, or a hospital, it's almost like a fancy hotel! And you know what? I absolutely love having you here and I'm going to miss you terribly when you leave because you're such a fun person to be around!"

Maria had taken in her beautiful surroundings, which did look like a lovely hotel, and she felt very flattered by my comments. I had given her a big hug when I told her that I would miss her when she left, so she had hope that she would return home soon. In the meantime, it really wasn't such a bad place to be after all. I would then redirect her mind from thoughts of leaving and "home" by walking with her to some activity that was going on in the facility and encourage her to join in. The requests to call her daughter to come and pick her up gradually subsided as she became more and more at home in our facility, and one day her daughter reported that as they drove up to the facility after an outing, her mother had commented to her, *"It's good to be home again."*

An alternative way to have handled her request might have been to simply begin to ask her questions about her home. Asking her where it was, what did it look like, how long had she lived there, and then gradually begin to lead the conversation onto a different topic. This can work well if you are able to take the time to engage them in a lengthy conversation, but I was usually in the middle of some project when Maria would come into my office. As I mentioned previously, it is not a "lie" to redirect people with dementia in this way. We call them "therapeutic fibs" because it is something they want to hear and it doesn't lead into arguments.

One man from the clergy whose wife has dementia, said during a support group meeting: *"Nowhere in the Bible does it say lying is a sin. It says we're not to bear false witness against our neighbor, but I believe there is a higher truth we need to hold to in situations such as this. You can tell the truth and hurt someone badly, or you can tell them something close to the truth to help alleviate their confusion or suffering."*

I feel this man is right. The truth is much too brutal and painful for a person with a damaged brain who no longer has the ability to understand reasoning, and who will forget the entire conversation in a short time anyway. Once we began to know more about our residents, we could more easily simply redirect the conversations away from their concerns without resorting to "therapeutic fibs." However, I feel strongly that if I'm that person with dementia who wants to go home, as long as you are treating me kindly with compassion, and maintaining my hope that I will get what I want, it doesn't matter to me if you're telling me a "therapeutic fib," or if you're talking circles around the topic. As long as you've replaced that worried look on my face with a smile, you've accomplished your goal of keeping me happy while maintaining my dignity.

I urge my client families to begin the facility search early and to get their names on the lists "just in case." They can always decline if a bed becomes available and they're not ready to admit their loved one. But it's far better to have done the legwork and the paperwork in advance, than to wait until a crisis forces them to place their loved one in any facility with an available bed.

Feelings of guilt and depression at having to place a loved one in a facility are always present in varying degrees, but guilt and depression never, ever contribute anything helpful to the immediate situation. They are a part of the grieving process as described by Dr. Elizabeth Kubler-Ross as denial, anger, bargaining, depression, and acceptance that we human beings go through with every major loss in our lives. The goal is to try to get through the stages with as little damage to ourselves as possible, and without getting stuck in any one stage for too long. Being unable to move out of one of those stages for extended periods of time (such as being depressed for years over an illness or event) calls for compassionate counseling in order to move on.

The next story tells about what happens to Sam and Minnie when the difficult decision is made for nursing home placement.

Forever Following

Sam and his wife, Minnie, had been high school
sweethearts and married right after graduation. They
raised three children, all of whom had married and now
lived in different states. When Sam was diagnosed with
Alzheimer's at the age of seventy-eight, Minnie vowed
she would care for him until the end. She was in fairly
good health for a seventy-seven year old woman, and
she was certainly determined, but friends and family
immediately saw that the biggest problem may be the
fact that Minnie weighed only about 105 pounds, while
Sam's weight was around 220. But, Minnie was not
easily dissuaded once she made up her mind, and she
refused to consider having any of the children move in
to help out.

Sam's descent into Alzheimer's was a slow one, and
after almost seven years of caring for him in their
home, Minnie's health was now compromised. She had
developed high blood pressure, her kidney function was
quickly declining, and she was in danger of developing
diabetes. Only when she fell and broke her wrist and
her arm while helping Sam into the house from the
backyard, did she tearfully agree that she could no
longer care for him at home. The decision was made to
place him in a nearby nursing home.

Sam was still able to walk slowly, but needed to
hold onto the person beside him or he would become
agitated and unsteady. When given a walker to hold

onto, Sam simply stood still and could not understand how to use it. Minnie said that for the past three years, Sam had been holding onto her and walking everywhere with her, and furthermore, if she walked out of his sight, he would become upset and attempt to find her while loudly calling her name. She said it then took her some time to calm him down, so she had simply taken him everywhere she went. That meant even when she went to the bathroom! In the kitchen, he would always try to "help" her out and would be just a step away, but always touching her at all times. When they went to bed, if she arose during the night to use the bathroom, Sam would awaken and go look for her and he often wouldn't go back to sleep. Her solution to that problem had been to drink very little liquids herself, so she wouldn't need to get up to use the bathroom at night. This solution had contributed to her current blood pressure and kidney problems.

Minnie was deeply depressed and felt guilty at having to put Sam in a nursing home, and she would take a bus to visit him several times a week. Her doctor and her family finally got her to agree to begin antidepressant medication and after several weeks, her depression started to lift. I believe that in addition to taking the medication, it was seeing Sam able to have a good quality of life in the nursing home that helped her overcome her guilt and depression.

Sam had always liked music and he also liked to look out the big picture window at the birds gathered around the bird feeder. He did occasionally follow staff around, but was content to stop following if they gave him a big hug and a smile and then engaged his mind in something he liked to watch or do. He never stopped following Minnie though, and would immediately attach himself to her arm when she appeared, and they would happily wander through the halls or sit and look out the windows together. When it was time for Minnie to leave, a staff worker would bring Sam his favorite snack and a big glass of milk, block his view of Minnie with his own body, and Minnie would make her exit without a fuss. She had become accustomed to giving him silent good-bye kisses before she actually left so she didn't upset him by saying the words. Sam's attention could easily be directed to something he enjoyed, and once Minnie was out of his sight for a few minutes, he would forget about her having been there.

Sam did have a good quality of life in that nursing home. He had forgotten years ago that he had Alzheimer's, and as long as he was not being asked to do something he disliked (such as take a bath), he was pleasant, cooperative, and happy.

Minnie continued to struggle with her depression and guilt for a period of about two years before she was able to let it go. She told me once during our many talks that it felt as though half of her had literally been ripped away from the side of her body when Sam had to be admitted to the facility. That constant presence in her life and on her arm of the man she loved was suddenly gone. Yes, I could see how she felt, and it was a different kind of grief than what she experienced from watching Sam succumb slowly to Alzheimer's. There are so many good-byes in dementia, and none of them are easy.

Old Glory

Bobby was a World War II Veteran who was admitted to our facility and who reminded me so much of my father. He would rather be dead than be there, and he battled depression because of wanting to be home. Despite these painful feelings, Bobby had a sharp wit and a wonderful sense of humor and we tried to capitalize on that at every opportunity.

His dementia progressed and he declined quickly from a fairly robust man who knew what "E-X-I-T" meant, and who could also read and understand the sign on the locked exit door which read "Press bar and door will unlock after 15 seconds." It was only a matter of months until he could walk only with the assistance of a walker, and even that was difficult for him. He pretty much forgot about constantly wanting to go home as his world became smaller and smaller, and he became more content.

As with all residents in facilities, it was crucial for us to maintain Bobby's dignity, treat him with respect, and honor him for the wonderful person he was.

It was Veterans Day and our facility was having a party with a program to honor the handful of vets who lived with us there. We had told Bobby about the program, but he really couldn't quite grasp what we were talking about. His damaged mind had lost the meaning of most of those words.

All the residents and staff were ready in the gathering room when the local VFW arrived to give the short program, and with rousing sounds of patriotic music being played, they marched into the room wearing their uniforms and carrying a large United States flag. I was holding the door open and I happened to glance over at Bobby and what I saw made my eyes fill with tears. Bobby had one hand on his walker and was struggling to stand erect from his chair while at the same time holding his right hand in a shaky salute as the flag he fought for on foreign soil so many years ago appeared before him. A staff person nearby also saw his struggle to stand and quickly stepped up to support him while he maintained his salute until the music ended. Now he understood, now he remembered. The sight of the flag and the sound of the music found the area of his brain that was still intact and the connection was made.

It was painful and it was profound to watch, and when I gave Bobby a hug afterwards (for my sake as much as for his sake), I could see the tears he had shed during the short program. *"That was nice,"* was all he could manage to say, and what a wonderful hug he gave me.

I'm so thankful for this special memory Bobby gave me. These many years later, this story still has the ability to bring tears to my eyes as I tell it or write about it.

"C'mon--Give Us A Hug"

That's what this happy little lady would always say when she saw me or anyone else come into the nursing home hallway where she sat in her wheelchair. I was always glad to comply and she was a great hugger! It always put a smile on both our faces.

I never made time to stop and visit with her because I was there to visit a friend and didn't want to take any time away from that, but in looking back, I now regret that I didn't get to know her better. I'm not even sure of her name because she told me several different names, so I just called her "Sweetie" and that seemed just fine to her. I assumed that she had some type of dementia since she never seemed to recall that I had just given her a hug on my way past her, and also because she had changed her name on me at least three times. She didn't appear to be able to use a wide range of words either, so I smile when I think of how she compensated for that lack by coming up with, "C'mon, give us a hug."

You may recall that I said earlier in this book to never underestimate the power of your smile and gentle touch and I know that many elders, whether they have dementia or not, begin to experience what I call "skin hunger." They've lost their spouse, their children may not be a daily presence in their lives, they're old, and possibly a bit crotchety at times. They get very few hugs in their lives now, and when anyone does actually touch them, it's only to help them dress, undress, or get out of a chair. They develop a real hunger for a compassionate touch from another person: a touch that says, "I'm so glad you're with me right at this moment in time."

There are people who have never been comfortable giving or receiving affectionate hugs, and I've had several families tell me they're surprised at seeing their loved one accepting and appearing to enjoy hugs from the staff because they've "never been one to show affection like that." Maybe when the area of the brain that controls their social graces becomes damaged, they're able to forget whatever it was that kept them from wanting to give and receive affection from others. That can become such a gift to adult children of a parent who had lived their entire lives with this reserved and undemonstrative person, and who now find that same parent giving them warm and loving hugs or wanting to hold their hand when walking with them.

I used to tell my staff to hug residents often because every time you put a smile on their faces, you've helped to brighten their day as well as your own. We would even occasionally have "hug contests" to see which resident would give the most hugs to staff. What happy, calm days those were for everyone! So go ahead and give us a hug!

"He Won't Keep His Shoes On!"

"He allows me to put his shoes on, but two minutes later he takes them off again, then sometimes he puts them back on, then he takes them off again! What are we supposed to do to keep his shoes on?"

The very exasperated, young aide was in my office in a quandary about how to keep Junior from taking his shoes off and walking around the facility in his stocking feet.

"Have you checked his feet to see if he has a sore anywhere, or checked to see if there is something wrong with the shoes?"

"Yes, and I even tried different shoes and slippers, but he still keeps taking them off. He denies any pain but I can't figure out what the problem is."

"Okay, after breakfast, bring Junior here to my office and I'll check him over and talk to him."

There wasn't a red or tender spot to be seen on Junior's feet, and I asked him if his shoes fit okay.

"Yeah, these are okay."

"Junior, do you have other shoes that are not okay?"

"Oh no, I like them fine, but I can't use them."

"Use them for what?"

"Well, I don't know, you know, I--I--I don't know."

"Okay, Junior, it's not a problem, I was just curious. Do you just like to walk around in your stocking feet sometimes?"

"Well, yeah, don't you?"

It seemed quite possible that Junior had the thought that he wanted to walk around in his stocking feet so he removed his shoes, and then as he carried his shoes around, he forgot the initial thought. Since he had his shoes in his hands he then decided to finish getting dressed and put them back on. This behavior continued for a few weeks, and I assured the staff and Junior's wife that it would likely resolve on its own and that it was okay if he wanted to walk around in his stocking feet. We would just need to be sure to check that he had clean socks on at all times.

The behavior did disappear after awhile, and it's now one of the little things I think about when Junior comes to mind, and I miss him and his stocking feet all over again.

I always tell staff and families that no matter what the behavior is that's driving you crazy today, it will disappear as the dementia progresses, and there may actually come a day when you wish for that behavior back again.

Living or working with people who have dementia can be likened to being stuck on a boat in the middle of unpredictable seas, and the captain at the helm is a five-year-old tyrant. Sometimes you love him for the sweet person he can be, and other times you find yourself plotting to throw him overboard. You never know when the seas will rise up against you, and you certainly never know when the small tyrant will decide to have a temper tantrum. Frustration is always so very close at hand when you are living or working with people who have dementia. Things just don't stay done, and the people with dementia just don't stay the way you left them five minutes ago. The rules of the game seem to constantly change for the caregiver and when you're feeling stressed by lack of sleep or the pressure to get tasks accomplished, there are times when you just wish you could stop playing the game. You need a break; you need frequent breaks away from the frustration and the stress. Otherwise it will just keep building in you until it destroys your health, your job, and your relationships. When you're regularly experiencing this type of stress, it is most assuredly perceived by your loved one with dementia, and in turn has a negative affect on them. Even though they are not able to figure out the reasons for the tension, they will reflect it back to you in their behavior which results in even more challenges for you.

When you are a caregiver of people with dementia in a facility, my fervent hope is that you love what you're doing and you love people with dementia, otherwise the challenges you encounter daily in your duties will make you hate your job, and ultimately resent those elders whose quality of life *(whose very lives)* depend upon your caregiving abilities. It becomes crucial to have the ability to go with the flow, to acknowledge that there will always be disruptions to your day, to your schedule, and going with the flow helps immensely in preventing the little things from becoming major frustrations. That's always much easier said than done, and it has to become a way of thinking, of being, when you're with people with dementia. Even then, there will be times when you need to get off that boat and away from that little "tyrant."

Unique Problems When The Husband And Wife Both Have Dementia

Randall and June were a married couple living in our dementia-dedicated assisted-living facility. They both had dementia, but Randall also had Parkinson's Disease and was confined to a wheelchair. They lived in a suite of rooms at the end of the hallway and you would rarely see one of them without the other. June would push Randall in his wheelchair about the facility wherever he wanted to go, and she wouldn't hesitate to jump up and attempt to see to his every need.

One evening the staff person assigned to that area called me to complain that she had assisted Randall and June in getting their pajamas on and into bed three times now, and that every time she returned to check on them, she found that June had gotten Randall up and was in the process of getting him dressed again. June obviously felt it was time to get up and get dressed, and Randall was understandably becoming a bit short-tempered by then. He was yelling at her and she was yelling right back at him, but still continuing to help him out of his pajamas. This fourth time, another staff person took June out to a quiet area and gave her some hot chocolate while Randall was again prepared for bed.

Since this was an obvious deviation from June's normal level of confusion, I suspected a urinary tract infection, and my suspicions were confirmed when we tested her urine. We quickly got the order to start an antibiotic, and made sure she was feeling tired before we returned her to her room. We verbally reinforced with her many times that it was bedtime, and when we quietly entered their rooms again, June saw that Randall was sleeping peacefully and she settled into her own bed. June quickly responded to the antibiotic and returned to her old self again in a very short time, but until she did, it was a challenge for the staff to keep her from upsetting Randall with her constant fussing over him.

Because of their deeply engrained routines established in our facility, a whole new set of problems developed for June after Randall passed on. We had a discussion with the family about how to tell June of his passing, and they decided they would tell her, take her to the viewing and the funeral, and then after that, if she asked where he was, would make up a story that he would be back shortly. The family felt they didn't want her to be re-oriented every day to the fact that he had died, and become brokenhearted all over again every time, and we agreed. We all felt June would readily accept the explanation that Randall was "at the doctor's office."

The family reported that June held up well at the viewing and the funeral. There were a few times when she forgot why she was with all these people and where they were, so they then reminded her Randall had died. Naturally she cried and was very sad, but overall she did well and was able to say good-bye to her husband of many years at the appropriate time.

The staff at the facility made it a point to give June hugs literally every time they were near her because we all knew that on some level, in her damaged brain she knew she was suffering, that something important to her was missing, and she would derive much comfort from many warm hugs and smiles, and it worked both ways. We would miss Randall, too, and it was as therapeutic for us to give the hugs and smiles, as it was for June to receive them.

June was so accustomed to taking care of Randall that after he passed away, she could be found pushing an empty wheelchair and talking to Randall as if he were still in it. We knew we would have to move her to a private room because she would believe that anyone in Randall's bed would either be Randall, or an intruder. The family agreed to the proposal, and June was not opposed to it, so we moved her to a single room in another hallway. A problem arose when she continually remembered to go to her old room, which we kept locked while vacant, and she would become upset when she couldn't get the door open. We decided to leave the door unlocked, made up the beds, and when we couldn't find June in her new room, we knew we could likely find her sitting in the rocker in her old room. June made fewer and fewer trips to the old room as the days went by until she accepted the new room as her own and she forgot about her old room and Randall's constant presence at her side.

"I've Had Two Of The Best Things Happen To Me Today."

Humor is as essential in the workplace as it is in the home when you're dealing with dementia. Here's my favorite humorous story about Al.

Al liked to come into my office and just sit in the visitor's chair from time to time, especially if he saw several people in there with me since he liked to be in the middle of people. He was usually quite happy and pleasant and loved it when we would chat with him and give him hugs.

Aimee was a beautiful, young woman who was working in our facility as a summer intern in management, and she always brightened a room when she entered it. Al would just beam when Aimee would give him a hug, and he would always compliment her and tell her how lovely she looked.

One morning after Aimee gave Al a big hug, he told her and the rest of us standing there in his slow, western-type drawl: *"Well, now I've had two of the best things happen to me today."*

"What are those two things, Al?"

"The first one was I had a good bowel movement this morning, and the second one was that nice hug I just got!"

152

From that day forward, we never let Aimee forget that she ranked second to a bowel movement!

"...I'm Just So Embarrassed..."

"Oh, I'm just so embarrassed, and I'm so sorry you have to help me with this! I just don't know what happened!"

This is what Janey would say to us every time we found her in the bathroom attempting to toilet herself. She still knew where the bathroom was, and still knew when she had to go, but the mechanics of getting her clothing down, and properly using the toilet paper were now beyond her abilities, and she always required our help. It was so important to maintain her dignity because she was truly embarrassed by her need for our help with such a private function.

"Don't be embarrassed, Janey. That's why we're here. We can help people when they need it."

"Well, I'm glad you're here since I don't know what I would have done!"

"I'm glad I was here too, Janey. I really enjoy being helpful."

We quickly discovered that Janey became even more embarrassed if a male attendant tried to assist her in the bathroom. Try to imagine yourself today in that situation. You're in a bathroom and you have managed to smear feces all over you, your clothes, and the toilet. You can't figure out how to get it off, and then in walks a young man who says he's there to help you. Personally, I would find it embarrassing enough to have a young woman come to help me in that situation. I would be mortified if a young man were to do the same.

Keeping that in mind, we would always attempt to keep an eye on Janey, and if she wasn't around, we would send a female resident into the bathrooms to look for her. A toileting schedule was of little help to her because her prolapsed uterus exerted a constant pressure on her bladder, and she had lost every pessary (a device to keep the uterus from pressing on the bladder) they had inserted to correct that problem. She would always go into the bathroom thinking she needed to urinate, but then end up many times having small bowel movements and wiping, wiping, wiping with only two small squares of toilet paper. It seems many elders who lived through the Depression had that habit of using very small amounts of toilet paper. You're certainly never going to get them to change that habit, so it's best if you try to establish a toileting schedule, and calmly and gently assist them in the clean-up process. Knowing this person with dementia is going to completely forget about their embarrassment in the entire episode can be comforting to the caregiver, until the next time.

The most important thing is to maintain the dignity of the person with dementia and act as if it's not a burden in any way for you to help them.

Sometimes humor can help in embarrassing situations such as this, but you really have to have a good idea ahead of time if that might be the case.

Bathroom Humor

Eunice had a very sharp wit and a great sense of humor, and she was having a lot of trouble having a bowel movement. She was impacted, again, and it was my duty to put gloves on and using copious amounts of Vaseline, manually remove the impaction.

She had been sitting on the toilet for some time attempting to push the fecal material out, but it was stuck, so the staff sent for me. When I walked into the bathroom with my gloves, Vaseline, and a cheerful, "Hello," Eunice took one look at me and grumbled, *"That's easy for you to say."*

Knowing she would understand the humor in my comment, I replied, *"Eunice, do you realize that this is the highlight of my day?"*

"Oh, you poor thing, you. That's bad!" she responded.

Eunice was also the person who one day was in a bit of a grumpy mood, when I gave her an impromptu little back scratch. She grudgingly said, *"Thank you, that felt good."*

I then held my hand out and said, *"That will be a quarter, please."*

Eunice replied with a snort, *"Huh! Good luck getting that,"* and off she went.

When it works, humor will be one of the best tools you have to help calm and redirect a person with dementia. It helps them feel "normal" again when they can "get it" and laugh along with you. If it falls flat and they just don't "get it," then you just move on to the next topic.

The Patient's Perspective: Where Are These Thoughts Coming From?

In earlier stories in this book, I talked about how important it is to get out of your own reality and into the reality of the person with dementia to understand where they're coming from and you can then redirect their thoughts and actions. This is a vital skill that must be learned by workers in facilities, as well as by family members in the home. That goal of keeping the person with dementia happy, safe, and healthy, with dignity could never be met unless you were willing to go into that person's damaged brain and help them find a safe way through their confused thoughts.

Of course knowing the personality and past of this person is extremely important for caregivers, but it's most important to know what makes that person calm or what makes them upset _now_ in their dementia when they can't verbalize what it is that's causing their discomfort.

I recall several gentlemen in the late stages of dementia in various facilities I worked at who would become agitated and strike out every time a caregiver attempted to toilet them by pulling their pants down. The obvious trigger for the agitation in these cases was the act of pulling the pants down and since the person couldn't say, "STOP THAT, I DON'T WANT YOU TO DO THAT..." they reacted in the only way they could to stop it. They struck out at the person who was trying to help them.

Because these gentlemen had lost the ability to understand the spoken words, there was no way the caregivers could make them understand what was going on or the need for the intrusion, so it was vital that the caregivers knew this was the reaction they could expect and take steps to avoid injury to themselves and to the person with dementia. A key part of that was to maintain a calm and gentle demeanor at all times while continually reassuring the person. Let me illustrate one way two staff members could safely toilet a man named Sherman: *"Hi, Sherman. I would like you take a short walk with me now."*

They are making eye contact, smiling, and holding out their hands to him to help him stand up from the chair. Since their body language says "friendly, nice, happy" even if he doesn't understand a single word of what they're saying, he agrees and takes their hands and walks into the toilet area.

One staff person faces Sherman, takes both his hands in hers, makes eye contact, and with a smile in her voice as well as on her face says: *"Sherman, we are going to take that wet brief off of you now and put a clean, dry one on. It will only take a minute and we'll be very gentle."*

The second staff person begins to pull his pants down and Sherman immediately becomes agitated and attempts to "box" the person holding his hands. She maintains her hold on his hands, maintains eye contact, and in a soothing, calm voice repeats over and over: *"Sherman, it's okay. We're almost done. Sherman, it's okay..."*

The second person is quickly removing the wet brief, wiping him with <u>warm</u> wipes, and replacing the brief. Sherman could never understand why people he didn't know were doing these things to him and he would always react by striking out to make them stop. Knowing he would react in this way, and preparing in advance for it, kept him and the staff safe.

I was the recipient of Sherman's agitation one morning when I was helping to get the residents up and dressed for breakfast. I knew he became upset during toileting, so another staff person assisted me with that. Then I seated Sherman on his bed, fully clothed, and kneeled in front of him to put his shoes on. As soon as I tightened the shoelaces, Sherman grabbed a fistful of my hair. As painful as that was, I maintained my calm, moved toward him slightly so he wasn't pulling any more, and slowly moved my face up to make eye contact with him. I smiled at him and gently took his hand from my hair. Thankfully, he let go of my hair to take my hand and I realized I had likely caused him pain in some way while tying his shoe. I replaced the shoes with slippers (while keeping my head out of range) and made a mental note to speak to the rest of the staff to see if they had had this problem with him as well. It turned out that nobody had that experience with Sherman before or after that. It was just something about the way I did it that upset Sherman that morning.

You'll often never be able to figure out why a person with dementia acts or reacts in a certain way, but it's imperative to remember that *your reaction to them* is what will determine the outcome of every encounter. So, seeing the situation from their perspective will help guide your reactions to keep you both safer.

"...Something Terrible Has Happened To Them..."

I was walking down a hallway in the dementia facility where I worked when I glanced into Myra's room, and saw her sitting on her bed sobbing. I went to her, sat beside her, and put my arm around her because I knew how much she liked to be hugged: *"Myra! What's wrong? Tell me, why are you crying?"*

"I just know something terrible has happened to them. They're not here yet!"

"Who is not here yet, Myra?"

"My husband and the babies! He said they would come here, but they're not here and I just know something terrible has happened to them!"

She began to sob even louder and I knew she was likely referring to the twins she had given birth to many years ago who died in infancy, as well as her husband who had passed away some time ago.

"Oh, Myra, (hugging her harder) I'm so sorry you're upset by this. I would be upset too, but you know what? I'm going to go right now and make some phone calls to see just where they are and why they're not here yet. I want you to dry those tears and I'll be back in just a few minutes. Okay?"

"Okay. You find them."

I left the room and simply waited around the corner for a few minutes while listening to what she was doing. She had stopped crying and was just sitting and waiting. I knew that her short-term memory had deteriorated but that she would remain upset unless I gave her some reason not to be upset. I entered the room with a smile and a happy expression.

"Great news, Myra! Your husband called and left a message at the front desk. The car had a flat tire and he has to fix it, but then he and the babies will be here to pick you up. I'm so sorry you didn't get that message earlier, Myra."

"Oh!" (She gives a huge sigh of relief.) *"That is good news."*

"It sure is. I have a great idea, Myra. Why don't you come with me and while you're waiting for them to get here you can help your friends out in the kitchen. I just passed by there and I see they're getting ready to bake something, and I've eaten some of your wonderful baking!"

I tucked her arm in mine and we walked toward the resident kitchen where the activity director was assisting a group of residents with baking holiday treats. I was told Myra had declined to participate in this activity earlier, but I felt she would now be willing to join in.

Myra and I had been chatting along the way to the kitchen about some of her favorite things to bake, so by the time we arrived at the kitchen and she was welcomed into the group, she had already forgotten about her husband and the babies. She was back to her laughing, happy self.

I think as she had been sitting alone in her room, something had triggered thoughts of those babies she lost so many years ago and she became trapped in that sadness. She would have remained trapped there had I not happened to "rescue" her from those thoughts. I was able to successfully talk her out of that mood by first acknowledging that she certainly had a right to be upset. I didn't tell her she was being silly to think those thoughts, and I certainly didn't try to re-orient her by reminding her that her husband and babies had all died a long time ago. If I had made that mistake, Myra would have reacted in one of two ways: (1) She would have believed me and cried even harder, mourning their loss all over again while berating herself for forgetting they had died; (2) She would have accused me of lying to her and may have even struck out at me for telling her such an awful lie. Neither one of those reactions are desirable from any person with or without dementia. Re-orienting Myra to the fact that her family was dead would serve only to torture her. Instead, I chose to tell her a "therapeutic fib" that I knew would get her brain off of that very sad subject and redirected onto something pleasant.

As I mentioned before, I don't advocate automatically lying to people with dementia, but when the situation calls for it and you can't quickly think of a way to talk around a subject (such as this very emotional one) then reassuring them by getting into their reality and changing the outcome will usually relieve their anxiety.

In Myra's mind, I had just given her back her beloved husband and babies, safe and sound, and she was happy again.

"YOU DRUNKEN BASTARD!"

Sometimes it's difficult to tell if people with dementia are creating new stories for their past lives, or if they are pulling together bits and pieces of their lives and the lives of friends and family. It doesn't really matter where the stories are coming from, but what does matter is that you treat that story as if it is their own and recognize the feelings they are experiencing in that moment.

You'll recall Bea from some previous stories where I mentioned just how feisty she was and how she would fight for what she believed. In this story, Bea believed another resident, named Bill, was her husband Philip, and would never be convinced otherwise. Just to test it out, one day our director decided to see how deeply engrained Bea's belief was. Bea and Bill were both in her office and when Bea called Bill "Philip," the director said, *"Bea, do you realize that this man's name is Bill? It's not Philip and he's not related to you at all?"* Even though Bill had shaken his head in the affirmative when she made that statement, Bea looked from one to the other, then walked over to Bill, put her hand up in front of her mouth and said in a loud whisper to Bill: *"She thinks your name is Bill!"*

Bea and Philip had been married for a long time before he died and left her a widow out on the farm. Their one daughter had married and was living nearby, and Bea managed for many years living alone in the big farmhouse. It was heart wrenching for the daughter when she had to place her mother in our facility because she could no longer function safely alone at home.

It wasn't long after her admission to our facility that Bea began believing that Bill, another resident in the facility, was her husband Philip. Because Bea was so small, had very straight, short, white hair and walked with a limp, Bill saw her as a young boy. So, he never minded it when she came up to him and took his hand and began walking everywhere with him, but we had to devise ways of separating them when it was time for bed, or when Bill's wife would come to visit.

Bea and Bill got along very well and roamed all over the facility holding hands and occasionally chatting, except for those few times when Bea would decide that Bill, who she now believed was Philip, had been out drinking and was now drunk: *"You bastard! You've been out drinking all night again, haven't you?"*

"What are you talking about? I haven't been drinking!"

"Don't you lie to me again. I know when you've been out whoring around and getting drunk! Don't think you can hide it from me for one second!"

Staff would have to intervene and rescue poor Bill because he couldn't figure out why someone would treat him so badly when he wasn't even drinking. We would just tell him that she thought he was somebody else and she had made a mistake and keep them separate for awhile until Bea forgot about it. In order to get Bea away, we usually did it by telling her the baby needed her, and then distract her until she calmed down and her mind went elsewhere. It always helps to know ahead of time what distraction will be most successful with any person with dementia.

When Bill's wife came to visit, we would put out the word over the walkie-talkies that she was approaching in order to give staff time to locate Bea, and if necessary, separate her from Bill before he saw his wife. We knew he would hurry across the room to hug and kiss her and we also knew if Bea saw that, she wouldn't hesitate to literally fight for her "husband." Bill's wife was aware of the situation and would take steps to ensure they wouldn't run into Bea in the facility as they walked around. She was glad Bill had a friend to keep him company throughout the days, and we knew nothing sexual would occur between Bea and Bill because Bill thought Bea was a young boy. He always called her "Picklepuss," and he took great comfort in her company.

Eating Everything In Sight!

Charlie was a gentle giant of a man who had started showing signs of Alzheimer's when he was in his fifties. It was fortunate that he remained a sweet, gentle soul until he passed on, because he was just so big, he could have caused injuries to a number of people in the process of his daily care.

In Charlie's current world, food was everything. He would put just about anything into his mouth thinking it was something to eat. As you can imagine, this posed quite a challenge to us in the facility because Charlie was still quite mobile and seemed to see just about anything as edible. He wouldn't hesitate to break off a flower or two from a bouquet on a table and pop them into his mouth as he passed by. It didn't matter to him if they were real flowers or silk flowers! The one thing he refused to put into his mouth was his false teeth. He would politely hand them back to you, or even helpfully assist you to place them into your mouth.

One day Charlie was walking past a group of residents who were playing some type of game that involved pennies. He stopped and observed for a few minutes, then casually walked over and helped himself to a handful of pennies which he promptly popped into his mouth and began to chew. When I arrived, he was still chewing the pennies and either couldn't understand my requests to spit them out, or he didn't want to give them up. I had no choice but to try to fish them out with a gloved hand. Calmly and gently, I removed eleven pennies from Charlie's mouth and replaced them with a sandwich he quickly gulped down.

It was fortunate that he didn't resist my efforts as much as he could have because it's not uncommon for a person with dementia to clamp their mouth shut and refuse entry of anything. Charlie would gently push my hand away after each penny or two that I managed to snag, and I was quite relieved that he didn't bite me, even without his teeth in place.

Being the gentle soul that he was, Charlie also loved animals, dogs in particular. Every time he would see a dog someone had brought into the facility, he would drop to his knees, and looking like a big overgrown boy, allow the dog to cover him with kisses while he cried tears of happiness.

One day the local SPCA brought nineteen puppies to our facility for the residents to cuddle and play with, and when Charlie was led into the room, he got the biggest grin on his face and immediately threw himself down on the sofa (taking up the entire sofa as he stretched out) and patted his chest to indicate we should place a puppy on his chest. We put three puppies on Charlie's big chest, and I think all of us cried tears of happiness right along with him as he gently cradled and kissed them.

Animals can touch a part of a damaged brain that nothing else seems to reach, and the joy that can bring to both the person with dementia and the families is priceless.

Keeping people with dementia safe at home or in a facility is such a huge and constant challenge, and harm can come to them in ways you may never think of, such as Charlie swallowing any item he put into his mouth. We did manage to keep Charlie safe during his time with us, and I like knowing we also enriched his life by providing him with many of the things he loved best such as puppies to cuddle.

"Bea--Please Come Down Off That Fence..."

Whether they are in their own home, or in a facility, keeping the person with dementia from walking away to "go home" or "going to work" is just another type of challenge to all caregivers. This is another story of Bea and her early days in the facility with us which was just a glimpse of the ways in which this tiny, feisty lady would challenge us as caregivers.

When the door shut behind her daughter, Bea turned around and it was then that she realized she was going to have to stay in this facility with us. She was furious with her daughter for "dumping" her at our facility and cursed her for hours after she left. Bea then began to try to figure out how to "escape" to go back home where she belonged. The staff and I were attempting to "watch" her without appearing to do so, and we had finally managed to convince her to sit down to rest a bit just before dinner.

We had a lovely outdoor courtyard in this facility that was surrounded by a six foot high wooden fence, and had a 1 x 4 inch board running the entire length of it at about the 3½ foot level for stabilization.

Bea was waiting and watching, and the minute our attention was elsewhere, she was out into that courtyard. Even though Bea was only about four feet high herself, when we found her after only a few minutes of searching, she was already standing on that board, holding onto the top of the fence while trying to figure out how to get over it.

"Bea! What are you doing up there?"

"What's it look like I'm doing? I'm goin' home!"

"Bea, please come down off that fence. That's not the best way for you to get home."

She was not at all happy that I had discovered her. Since she couldn't maintain her precarious toehold on the 1 x 4 inch board for long, she finally allowed me to help her safely down.

That little exercise had expended much of her angry energy, and she calmed down enough to eat a small dinner, but to this day, I don't know how she managed to even get up there! The only thing I can figure out is that because she only weighed around eighty pounds, the bushes in front of the fence held her weight just long enough for her to get up on the board. She's the only person who ever got that far in their attempt to get over the fence, and I think the very fact that she was so small is what allowed her to get up on that board, but it was also what prevented her from getting over the top. She just wasn't tall enough to even see over the top!

Why Is Hydration So Crucial?

I can't stress strongly enough how important it is for caregivers to ensure that people with dementia stay adequately hydrated, and people with dementia are not at all concerned about it. If you ask them if they want something to drink, they often say they just had a drink and they're not thirsty. What you need to know is that the thirst mechanism in their brain may not be functioning correctly (and even if it is) they may not be able to interpret what that signal means anymore.

I would like to give you an idea of just what can happen if any elderly person is not adequately hydrated, and thus is dehydrated:

- Skin integrity is lost which will result in poor healing of wounds, rashes, skin tears, and a much greater chance of decubitus ulcers (bed sores) if they are immobile for any length of time.

- Constipation and/or obstruction in the bowel due to the lack of water helping to move the waste products through the colon. So many elderly people have bowel problems anyway (and when you add dementia to the picture) their chances of frequently suffering from constipation or obstruction increases greatly. Also, their ability to tell you about what is bothering them decreases with dementia, so trips to the ER are not uncommon for this problem.

- Increased chances for urinary tract infections. Because the urine becomes so concentrated from lack of water, and because hygiene is often compromised in people with dementia, their chances of developing a urinary tract infection (UTI) increases greatly.

- Increased confusion. That's just what they need! When you dehydrate a person with dementia even a little bit, their confusion increases.

- Medications will not be metabolized properly. When the kidneys don't have enough water to do their job, medications will not be broken down and metabolized properly so more of the medication will be excreted rather than utilized by the body as intended. When you consider that people tend to lose some kidney function as a result of aging, it becomes even more imperative to ensure they have adequate fluids to assist the kidneys to do their job.

- Increased risk for falls. Eventually people with dementia will fall because their brain is beginning to forget how to walk. Dehydration will contribute to increased confusion which will lead to an increased risk for falling. Even with mild dehydration, the brain is having more trouble than usual trying to make sense of what is going on around them.

When you look back at this list of very serious things that can happen to an elderly person just because they're not drinking enough fluids, I hope it motivates you to look for creative ways to encourage your loved one to consume more liquids.

Here are some hydration tips that have worked well for me in my day-to-day interactions with those wonderful elders with dementia:

- Keep them calm and happy. Sounds simple, but I'm sure you're already aware of just how difficult that can be. What you need to remember is that the happier and more calm they are, the more willing they will be to go along with whatever it is you want them to do. Let them be right, don't argue with them. If they say, "No, I just had my juice with my breakfast" and you know they haven't even had breakfast yet, rather than try to convince them they're wrong (again), saying something like, "Oh, I didn't realize you had already eaten. I'll just put this here in case you want to drink a little more." Put the glass on the table, urge them to sit down and "keep me company while I make myself some breakfast," and begin to talk about other subjects of interest while you prepare the meal. Then simply place the breakfast in front of them (all the while chatting about something else) and sit down with them and begin to eat. Chances are they will forget they had "already" eaten, and because you're eating, they will join you.

- This works well in a facility too, where you just invite the person to sit down for a cup of coffee (hot chocolate, tea, etc.) and "keep Mary and Joe company while they eat because you know how much they enjoy talking with you every morning." Then place the breakfast and drink in front of them when Mary and Joe receive their breakfast. If they still claim they have already eaten, simply say, "Oh, I'm sorry, I forgot. I can't take this back to the kitchen just now, so I'll let it sit here and pick it up later. Would you like some more coffee?" Often, when you look over a short time later, because Mary and Joe are eating, your reluctant resident will be eating and drinking also because it's a social situation, and as long as some of their social graces are still intact, they will follow along.

- The key is to not upset them by reminding them they're wrong. Any argument you enter into with a person with dementia will soon be forgotten by them, but you will carry it around for a long time! So, let them be right all the time (unless it's a safety issue like wanting to walk outside in the snow with no shoes on). Even then, it's not helpful to tell them they're wrong. You could simply follow them with the shoes until they realize they need them. Then you present the shoes and joke about how lucky it is that you thought to bring them!

- Keep favorite beverages on hand. They will be much more likely to drink fluids if what you're offering is something they enjoy drinking.

- Give them some control if possible. People with dementia have lost control over most of their lives and any time you can give them back some of that control, you will help them feel more "normal" and it will help calm them. Just think about all of the decisions you make on a daily basis. Now imagine someone else suddenly telling you you're wrong and you must do it their way. That's not "normal" for you and it's likely to upset you.

- In helping keep people with dementia hydrated, it's best not to give a choice that can be answered with a "No" answer such as, *"Are you thirsty? Do you want a drink?"* You can give them some control here by asking, *"Do you want some fresh iced tea, or some of that great lemonade I made yesterday?"* They don't have to decide if they're thirsty, they just have to focus on which flavor they prefer, but as the dementia progresses, even this simple choice is beyond their ability, and it's better to just present them with what you believe they prefer, and drink your own glass with them.

"I Want Beer!"

That was Mike's reply to us every time we asked him what he would like to drink. It didn't matter if we were asking at breakfast, lunch, snack, or dinner. He always wanted a beer. His family confirmed that he did drink beer daily, but it was not possible for him to have it in our facility because of the interactions with his medications. Mike wouldn't drink anything if he couldn't have beer, and because hydration is crucial for all the reasons I just mentioned, we handled this in the following manner: *"Boy, I'm not sure what kind of beer we have here, Mike. What kind do you usually drink?"*

"Miller, and not that weak stuff either."

"Okay, let me see what we have."

I bring him back O'Doul's "non-alcoholic" (0.5% alcohol) beer.

"Mike, I'm sorry but this is the only kind of beer we have right now. How about if you try this and we'll see how quickly we can get you some Miller beer?"

"I've never heard of this one, but I'll try it."

I pour him a glass and remove the bottle just in case he can read and understand "non-alcoholic."

Mike tried the O'Doul's and declared it "*almost not fit to drink*," but he did drink it at every meal and snack, and it kept him hydrated. Since his short-term memory was affected by the dementia, he would forget that we had had this conversation earlier in the day, and would always give the O'Doul's a try. We did continue to offer him other beverages, and eventually, as his dementia progressed, he began to stop asking for beer and began accepting juices and punches. I believe he had gone back in his mind to an age when he never drank beer, and that's when he began accepting other beverages.

Complimenting Gracie

Gracie would answer "no" to anything she hadn't thought of first. It didn't matter if it was wearing her favorite sweater, or drinking her favorite hot chocolate. If you asked her about it, she would automatically say "No." We knew that she was still a very social person who enjoyed being with others. Gracie also loved to look nice and be complimented, so we capitalized on those areas in order to get her to stay hydrated. Instead of asking her if she wanted a glass of water with her snack, we would approach her carrying two glasses and a pitcher of water and give her a big smile: *"Gracie! How beautiful you look this morning! Is that a new skirt you have on? I don't think I've seen that one before!"*

She would beam with joy at the compliment: *"Oh this old skirt? I've had this thing for at least a few years. No, it's not new at all."*

"Well, I think it just brings out the blue in your eyes in such a lovely way, and I think you should wear that skirt more often! I wish I had a knack for picking out beautiful clothing like you do."

During the time we're chatting about her clothing, and I'm complimenting her, I've simply handed her an empty glass, then the pitcher of water, and then I hold out my glass for her to fill. She is so focused on the clothing compliments that her social graces take over and she enters the "hostess in control" mode where she is serving me. We stand there and drink our water together as we continue to talk about clothing. She doesn't even realize she's drinking the water because the compliments about her clothing mean so much to her and she's focused on that.

This way of keeping Gracie hydrated could not work for long because the ability to "multi-task" or do anything simultaneously is lost fairly quickly with many types of dementia. Performing any task with the hands then requires great concentration and Gracie would not be able to chat about her clothing while pouring the water. Because she remained social for a long time, we were then able to simply place the beverage in front of her on the table and not mention it. When everyone around her began to eat and drink, Gracie followed along.

More Hydration Tips

Hydration is such a crucial part of keeping any person with dementia healthy and safe so I have included more tips on how to help them stay hydrated. These are critical tips to be utilized in facilities by the caregivers there as well as in every home by family caregivers:

- Give the person with dementia a large glass of water immediately upon awakening in the morning. This will be your best chance at getting them to drink an entire glass of water without a fuss. Recall how your mouth feels when you first arise in the mornings: like a platoon of soldiers has been marching through in muddy boots perhaps? These elders are no different and their mouths may be much drier because they often mouth breathe while they sleep. I suggest you enter the room, go into the bathroom and run a BIG glass of cold water (unless you know they prefer it warmer), set it on the nightstand and awaken them with a smile and a gentle touch. Assist them to sit up, hand them the glass, and then ask them which outfit they prefer to wear today. They will likely sit there and drink that entire glass of water while you are gathering their clothing and toiletries. You will be surprised at how much more alert they seem, how much better their balance is when they've started the day with a good dose of much needed water, and their kidneys are ecstatic!

- Give 4-6 oz. of water every time you give them medication. That little sip or two to just get the pills swallowed won't be enough for the kidneys to metabolize that medication. I used to tell my residents, "The doctor said you need to drink this whole cup of water with this medicine or it won't work right." They often grumbled about it, but they usually believed me and drank it. One day a woman said, *"Well then, let the doctor drink it because I don't want it!"*

- Beg, bargain, and plead with them to drink. I would tell my staff they could not feel as if they were above doing this because it's just so crucial to maintain hydration for these elders. Louisa just didn't like to drink anything, and every time you offered her a drink she would say, *"No, I don't want that."*

I would then say *"Please, Louisa, just one little sip? Would you take just one sip for me please?"*

"Oh, alright, just one."

I would give her a sip and then place the glass out of sight, chat with her for just 15-20 seconds since her short-term memory was quite poor, and then offer it to her again. We would go through the whole thing again and again until the entire glass of water was gone. As long as she thought she was just taking one sip as a favor to someone, she would do it.

- Sometimes bargaining works by saying something like, *"If you finish off this glass of water for me, then the least I can do for you is take you out to the garden after breakfast today."*

- Always give water with every snack. Every time food is offered, some beverage should also be encouraged (and not just "offered" to them) they need to be encouraged to drink it. This is especially important in facilities where snacks and drinks may be available at all times to everyone. A person with dementia doesn't have the ability to remember where they are, and often cannot interpret that "thirst" signal from the brain, or form the words to ask for a drink. People with dementia must be encouraged to drink multiple times daily.

- Always refill beverage glasses at meals with water when empty. This is important to teach staff to do in facilities and it's not something the staff will necessarily *want* to do because they are often in a hurry to get people out of the dining rooms. Many times a person with dementia will eat or drink something just because it's there in front of them, and even if it's only a swallow or two, that just helps keep them that much farther away from dehydration.

- Drink a glass of water with them. Many of us are walking around in a continual state of near dehydration and don't even know it. When you feel "thirsty" that's a sign that your kidneys already think there's a drought going on and have been calling for water from your other body cells. This is not a bad thing if there really is a drought going on, but it's causing you to have more wrinkles in your skin. You also don't have quite as much energy as you could, and your brain cells aren't firing at top speed because your body is diverting water to your kidneys. That's why the experts are all telling you to be drinking 6-8 glasses of water a day; something that is not all that easy to do unless you create a "habit" of doing it. If you can encourage an elder with dementia to drink a glass of water just by drinking one yourself, you're doing your own body a big favor too.

When you become committed to keeping a loved one hydrated, it becomes second nature to you after awhile. It becomes a habit; one of the most important ones you can develop.

Maintaining Weight Is Also Important

Right behind keeping people with dementia hydrated, comes the almost equally important topic of maintaining their weight.

Weightloss eventually comes to almost all people with dementia, and unless they started out obese, it's best to maintain their weight for as long as possible. Indeed, unexplained weightloss is now being seen as a predictor of some dementias, and can start to occur several years before any signs of the dementia. The following are some of the negative things that happen when elders, with or without dementia, lose a significant amount of weight:

- Their clothing won't fit properly and they can be walking along and suddenly their pants or skirt falls down. Aside from that being a dignity issue, it's certainly also a safety issue. They're just not as comfortable as they could be either. This could be what pushes that sweet little lady to go "shopping" in someone else's closet and she becomes a shrieking fighter when the owner of the clothing she's trying to wear attempts to take it back.

- Shoes no longer fit properly so they flop around on their feet causing sores and increasing their risk of falling, or they just keep taking them off and won't wear shoes.

- Dentures don't fit properly. In the facility this is where the person takes them out after a few bites of food (because they don't fit and it's uncomfortable to eat with them), wraps them in the paper napkin for safe-keeping, and the staff throws them away with the trash. Again, sore areas will be rubbed on the gums, and they just get tired of trying to eat with them in, so they stop eating and/or stop wanting to have the dentures in their mouth.

- "Malnutrition" is a word no facility wants to see in their charts, nor does a family wish to hear it applied to their loved one. Because these people often become so adamant about what, when, or how often they eat, the nutritional quality of the food they do eat may not be good enough to keep them from becoming malnourished.

- Poor skin integrity, and slow or no healing of wounds can be common, especially when they become malnourished. The skin is unable to remain intact with even the slightest bumps, and wounds take much, much longer to heal.

- Significant weight loss can contribute to an inability to fight off illnesses. When the body has to tend to just keeping a person up and moving it doesn't have the nutritional "strength" to fight off any of the viruses that are always around.

- If this person lives in a facility, then whatever department of the state that oversees what goes on in that facility will feel compelled to come in to visit to see just why this person has lost so much weight and just exactly what has been done to prevent it.

Stealing Cookies!

Joe was a thin, small man who never had much of an appetite, and when he came to our facility, at first he was despondent about being there, so he ate even less. Most of our attempts to cajole him into eating anything were unsuccessful. However, one day when I was walking through the hallway, I noticed the smell of fresh-baked cookies coming from the kitchen. I happened to see Joe sitting nearby and went up to him and whispered in his ear: *"Hey, Joe. Do you smell those cookies?"*

"Yeah, I believe I do."

"You know what? I have a key to the back door of the kitchen and if you'll come with me, we can snitch a couple of those cookies while they're still warm!"

"Okay!"

He did come with me to snitch a couple of those warm cookies and we devoured them right there in the hallway. I believe I had tapped into the mischievous little boy in Joe by sneaking in and getting the cookies. From then on, the kitchen would call my office to let me know when the just-baked cookies were on the cooling racks so Joe and I could make a cookie run multiple times a week! It helped Joe feel good, gave him some much needed calories, and it also made me start an exercise regimen to get rid of those cookie calories! I know for a fact that Joe would have refused those exact same cookies if I had offered them to him off the snack cart, so I felt fortunate to have found a way to help him enjoy some.

Tips To Help Maintain Weight

Here are some more tips on how to encourage people with dementia to eat, whether they are living in your home with you, or they are living in a facility, take these tips and use any or all of them to achieve your goal of keeping a person with dementia healthier and preventing weight loss:

- Maintain a calm, pleasant, and home-like environment. Studies have shown the less it looks like an institution, the better they will eat.

- At home, if the normal routine isn't working, try sitting in front of a picture window to eat, or maybe playing soft music in the background.

- Studies also show that having fish aquariums in the eating area helps people with dementia eat better. I'm pretty sure that wouldn't do much for me, but you do whatever works for them.

- Serve favorite foods. I was in a grocery store one day when a woman came by with a grocery cart being pushed by her husband, and the cart contained at least eight cartons of ice cream! She saw me looking at the cart and then at him. It was quite obvious to me that he had some type of brain impairment and she said with a little laugh, *"That's the only thing he'll eat!"* I replied, *"Good for you then for serving him what he wants!"* A balanced diet will likely be a thing of the past with these elders, so the priority changes to keeping them happy and fed.

- Serve one small dish at a time. This has been proven to be quite effective at getting people with dementia to eat better. Remember earlier when I talked about choices and how difficult it becomes for them to make even simple choices? When they're faced with a big plate or tray of food, they often automatically say, *"Oh no, I'm not hungry. Take it away!"* If you present one dish at a time, it's a much more achievable goal for them and they don't have to make those choices. In our facility when a resident sat down to breakfast, they had their juice, a cup of coffee or hot chocolate, and a small dish of fruit. When they finished the fruit, that dish was removed and they were served a jazzed up bowl of oatmeal with brown sugar, milk, and sometimes raisins. When they finished that, the bowl was removed and they were served a hot plate of something like bacon, eggs, and toast. And most of them ate it all!

- If you work in a facility where the food comes up to the floor on carts, make sure you only take off one dish at a time and in that case, the hot plate first.

- Milk shakes and/or high calorie/high nutrient supplement drinks if they refuse meals. As in the story with Joe, you can tap into that child within by offering them a good old-fashioned milk shake if they've refused a meal. Just be sure to wait a few minutes after their refusal so they "forget" they've said they weren't hungry.

- When I helped move my parents from one state to another, my father in the early stages of dementia, often refused to eat when we stopped. He just wasn't hungry. We simply went in and enjoyed our meal and ordered a chocolate milkshake and french fries "to go" and presented them to him on our return to the car. He always ate them and seemed pleased that we had thought to get them for him. I'm sure chocolate milk shakes will be the key to keeping me fed if I ever get dementia. You can always fortify those shakes by adding the supplement drinks, Carnation Instant Breakfast, or protein powder to them.

- Encourage your loved one to *"just have a cup of coffee."* Earlier when I spoke about hydration, I mentioned briefly about going along with their statement that they "already had breakfast/lunch/dinner," and just asking them to sit down and join you or others while you eat. We often had to do this every day for some residents who just had no appetite in the mornings. Even if they refused to do that, we would allow some time to pass, and then appear with the food and just place it in front of them as if it were the normal, routine thing to be doing. I can't count the number of times a resident, (and my father) told me they weren't hungry, but when the food was placed in front of them, they ate it all.

- Be sure the color of the dishes contrasts with the color of the food. Because people with dementia often have vision changes as the dementia progresses, they really cannot see white food on a white plate. Even a sandwich on a white plate is not necessarily "seen" by them. If your dishes are patterned, you may find the person with dementia trying to scrape up what they believe to be food when it's really the pattern on the plate. You'll save yourself and your loved one a lot of frustration by simply using inexpensive one-color plates and bowls. Blue is a good color since there aren't many blue foods.

- Don't force them to use utensils if they're having trouble with them. They may eventually "forget" how to use the utensils, and if you repeatedly attempt to "remind" them how to use them, you'll be in for a lot of very unnecessary battles and the result will be that they just don't eat.

- Sometimes if you "jump-start" the motion with the utensil, they can still use it. By that, I mean place the spoon in their hand and guide it into the food and then to their mouth. Sometimes the muscle memory then takes over and they can continue to eat using the utensil. Once they put it down though, you may have to jump-start the process again.

- Give "finger foods" when they can no longer use utensils or stay seated during meals. These are the foods they can pick up and eat as they walk around. Peas and mashed potatoes would certainly not be good choices here.

- You want to avoid hand-feeding an elder until you know they can no longer feed themselves because once you take over that task, their brain will forget how to do it. That means allowing them to eat with their fingers and hands if that's all they're capable of at that time: things like chicken tenders, large pieces of steamed vegetables such as broccoli or cauliflower, slices of fried or baked potatoes. If they're walking around while eating, they will often return to their plate for more, and if they don't, then you must continually supply them with the food as they walk.

- Try "sandwiching" foods when utensils can no longer be used. One woman in our facility no longer recalled what to do with the utensils at mealtimes and she absolutely refused to be fed. She would clamp her mouth shut and you couldn't get anything in. For some reason she also seemed unwilling to pick the food up with her fingers. One of the staff then discovered that if you placed any food in a slice of bread and handed it to her, she would eat it. From then on, she got delicacies such as spaghetti sandwiches, broccoli sandwiches·· whatever the menu called for that day, she received in a sandwich. She happily continued to feed herself in this manner, and she stopped losing weight.

- Assess for pain when a person with dementia stops wanting to eat. Janey was one of our residents who always had a great appetite, and when she could no longer feed herself, she allowed us to feed her. Then, over the course of a few days, she began refusing solid foods. She would drink all of her drinks, but would eat no solids. I asked her if anything hurt or if she had pain, and she denied either one. I then asked her if I could look in her mouth and when we removed her dentures I found a huge sore on her gums under her dentures. Sadly, this turned out to be a fast-growing and aggressive form of cancer, and I'm thankful she didn't linger long with it.

- Always think of pain, either acute or chronic pain such as arthritis, as a possible reason for a loss of appetite in a person with dementia. There have been studies in facilities done showing when they gave people with dementia Tylenol 3-4 times a day in addition to their regular medications, they were more social, they stayed out of their rooms more, engaged in more work-like activities, and they ate better. This says that at some level they were having chronic, nagging pain they weren't able to verbalize.

- Check to see if a new medication has been started. How many medications have the potential to upset your stomach? Almost all of them! And that person with dementia can't necessarily tell you, *"No, I don't feel like eating because I feel a little nauseated."* If a new medication has been started, and you suspect it may be causing some nausea, you should talk with the doctor to see if it might be short-term, or if they can switch to another dose or brand. If they are not taking a new medication, could one of their old medications be causing some stomach distress? You can ask the doctor if you can try something over-the-counter to help calm the stomach just to see if it helps. It's important to always ask the doctor because even simple antacids have the potential for causing more problems such as constipation or diarrhea and should be used sparingly. Possibly the distress has to do with excess gas, so an anti-gas medication used temporarily may help.

- Keep track of bowel movements. Another reason a person with dementia stops eating can be constipation and/or obstruction of the bowel. As distressing as this is to think about, and to actually keep track of for a loved one, it's essential information to have. The bowel often has problems with elimination as a person ages anyway, and when you add dementia to the picture where this person's eating habits have likely changed, you set the stage for repeated bouts of constipation or obstruction. When either of those hits, the person's desire to eat will probably disappear. The doctor will always want to know if bowel function is "normal" for this person when they are trying to assess for loss of appetite, increased confusion, falls, and a host of other problems that can come from a backed-up bowel. So knowing when this person last had a bowel movement, and whether it was a "normal" bowel movement for them is valuable information to be able to relay to the doctor.

Facility Caregiver Mealtime Tips

Now, for all those wonderful elders with dementia who are living in facilities, I have some tips for caregivers to enhance the dining experience for them. Families who have placed their loved one into such a facility can suggest these tips to help make life better for all of the residents in that facility. Remember, any time the residents are happy, the duties of the caregivers are made much lighter:

- Have assigned seating in dining rooms. Not only does this help caregivers easily determine if a resident is not present, it helps a resident maintain a sense of familiarity with their surroundings and the people around them. Often they cannot accurately know which specific seat is their assigned seat, but they still feel everything is familiar when they are there, and the more familiar you can make things for them, the calmer they will be.

- Placemats on the tables. Not only do they make the room look nicer, it helps define the boundaries at the table for the person with dementia. There will come a time as the dementia progresses, where the placemat is just something they think they can consume, but until that time, it's a positive addition to the dining experience.

- Seat higher functioning people with dementia away from people who need to be hand-fed. These higher functioning folks know this place isn't home and they don't especially want to be there. When they're forced to sit through every meal watching other people being fed, or eating with their hands, it definitely affects their appetite in a negative way. Instead, seat them together in a separate area if at all possible, where they can converse with one another, and have a "normal" dining experience. For quite awhile after she was admitted, Ella never wanted to go to the dining room because she thought her daughter was coming to pick her up to take her home "any minute now." We would tell Ella her daughter had left instructions for us to go ahead and provide a meal for her now, and her daughter would pick her up later after the meal. So Ella always thought she was eating in a "nice restaurant." She always wanted to know the name of it, and would often remark that she would like to come back to visit some time. Do you think she would have felt that way if she had had to watch people being fed, or eating with their hands?

- Discourage staff from mixing pureed foods together. There may come a time when that person with dementia requires a pureed diet because the brain is forgetting how to chew and swallow properly. When this happens, staff must remember this elder can still discern different flavors. They probably can't tell you what those flavors are, but they sure know if they like them or not! Just like an infant, they will spit out those foods they dislike. Try to imagine at your next meal that due to some dental surgery, your food has to be pureed. You have meatloaf, mashed potatoes, gravy, green beans, and slaw salad. Now imagine that your helper (mother, spouse, daughter, or son) is in a hurry, so they just glopped it all together into a bowl in order to save time and they start to shovel it into your mouth. Not only is this not appetizing in presentation or color, but do you even *want* to taste it? So if you see this happening in a facility, try to stop it so these elders can enjoy the distinct flavors of foods they like.

That was a lot of information that I feel is important for you to know, whether you are taking care of a loved one at home, or whether you are a caregiver in a facility. The more you know what that person likes to eat and drink, and the calmer and more comfortable you can make them feel, the better they will eat and drink. I'm positive this will also result in a sense of calm and comfort in you.

"I Have To Catch The Next Bus."

I was working in my office at the assisted- living facility to finish the staff schedule when Essie came to the doorway and asked: *"Excuse me, can you please tell me when the next bus stops here? I have to catch the next bus."*

"Oh, hello, Essie. Where are you off to today?"

"Why, I have to get home before my husband does. I have to get supper started."

"Well, Essie, the next bus doesn't stop here until noon, and I'll make sure I tell you when it's here so you won't miss it."

"Thank you so much!"

Off she went and I returned to my work. Five minutes later: *"Excuse me, could you please tell me when the next bus stops here? I need to catch the next bus."*

"Hi, Essie. The next bus won't be here until noon, and that's over an hour away. Why don't you find a comfortable spot on the sofa and I promise I'll tell you when it's here so you won't miss it."

"All right, thank you so much."

Off she went, and I again try to relocate my train of thought in the staff schedule. Five minutes later: *"Excuse me, but could you please tell me what time the next bus stops here? I really need to catch the next bus."*

I look up yet again to see her smiling face in my doorway and can't help but feel a bit impatient, and then I stop myself. Essie can't help that her brain is damaged and she can't remember this is the third time she's asked me the same question. If she could change I know she would, but she cannot, so I must be the one who does the changing. I must be the one who changes my attitude, my approach, and my priorities for her comfort and safety. I give her a big smile, rise from my desk and walk over to her:

"Are you anxious to get home, Essie?"

"Yes, I need to get dinner started for my husband."

"Well, you have plenty of time since the bus won't be here for over an hour. I promise I'll watch out for it and tell you when it's here." (I tuck my hand under her arm and we begin to walk toward the activities area while I continue talking.) *"Oh, look! They're painting beautiful pictures here! Essie, I know you have a lot of talent when it comes to painting. Why don't you sit down here and paint for awhile until the bus arrives? I promise you won't miss it!"*

Essie sat down with a smile and agreed to paint *"just one little picture."* I was confident that once she got her mind off that bus and engaged it in her painting, she would completely forget about needing to get dinner ready.

In my reality, there was no bus that stopped there, but I knew if I tried to orient Essie to my reality instead of getting into her reality, it would only confuse and possibly anger her. By entering her reality with her, reassuring her that I would help, and knowing that she would forget the entire scenario, I kept her calm, reassured her, and redirected her mind elsewhere.

That little sting of impatience should serve as a warning to anyone caring for a person with dementia. When you feel it, that's usually an indication that what *you're* doing isn't working, and *you* need to change your approach.

If I had taken the time to physically redirect Essie the first time she came to me, the next two interruptions would likely have been avoided. Any irritation and impatience I experienced needed to be directed at myself since I was the only party in this interaction who could effectively change the outcome.

"...You Have Such Beautiful Furniture!"

Lizzy was a tiny, very sweet, elderly woman with dementia who had become quite childlike in her speech and manners. Because I was smiling at her and touching her gently, she allowed me to draw blood from her arm, and as I carefully switched tubes, she reached up with her free hand to gently touch the Black Hills gold cross necklace I was wearing. She smiled and said, *"Oh, you have such beautiful furniture!"*

It was quite easy in this instance to understand that she meant "jewelry" instead of "furniture" but often it's not that easy when a person with dementia uses the wrong words. This inappropriate word usage has been called "word salad" and sometimes you have no idea what they are talking about. If that's the case, you should just respond to the emotion or the body language behind the mystery words. If they seem upset, give them a hug and you may try to offer simple questions such as "Are you upset?" or "Would you like some ....?" in order to try to figure out what is causing their distress. Many times, just the hug and the knowledge that someone cares is enough to help them feel calm and comfortable again.

The Thief Among Us

Esther is a short, hunchbacked little lady who almost always has a smile and a hug for everyone. She loves babies (dolls), and is usually carrying one around with her, along with at least one of her numerous pocketbooks, and possibly a magazine or two. Esther also happens to be a rather accomplished thief. When you're dealing with a person with dementia though, it's not thought of as stealing; it's called "shopping" or "borrowing."

I always knew to keep my desk cleared of extra pens, pencils, or notebooks when I would see Esther making her way toward my office. I've found it's always better to *prevent* having to get something away from a person with dementia, than it is to actually get it back, thus the attempts to keep my desk relatively cleared. Esther would stand in front of my desk and innocently ask me, *"How ya doin' today, honey?"*

She would calmly and slowly finger various items on my desk, and if she thought I wasn't looking, she would pocket those items and leave.

One day I stepped out of my office to use the bathroom and looked around for Esther. She was not in sight and I thought it was safe to leave my office door open and unlocked for a few minutes. When I returned, I discovered my appointment book, and the staff schedule I had been working on had disappeared. My first suspect was Esther, and sure enough, I saw her sitting on the sofa with them clutched against her breast along with a babydoll, and her pocketbook. I knew if I asked her to return them to me, she would not do so willingly, and would claim them as her own. She would become upset, possibly cry, or begin to curse me for trying to take her things. What I did instead, was knowing that she liked colorful items, I collected some magazines with bright pictures on the front, along with some unneeded papers destined for the recycle bin. I approached her with a big smile and said, *"Esther! Oh, thank you SO much (giving her a hug). You've found those papers I've been looking all over for them! Oh, I'm SO happy you found them. I'm almost finished with them so let me give you these papers to check for me while I finish those and then I'll give them right back to you."*

Esther eyed them for a moment, reached out for them, but still wouldn't release her hold on my items.

"Esther, I don't know how I would get all my work done without you to help me! You are so good at checking these papers for me. May I ask you to please look these over for me now, and then I'll get these other ones back to you shortly?"

Esther relinquished my items and took the proffered magazines and papers. I gave her a big hug and again thanked her for all her help. She felt good about "helping" me and I certainly felt good about getting my appointment book and schedule back without upsetting her.

Maintaining dignity and helping people with dementia feel valued are key things to remember when dealing with this population. Whether it's in a facility, or in your own home with a family member, using this approach will usually get you what you need while avoiding upsetting the person with dementia.

Read on for another wonderful story about Esther and her desire for other people's items.

Esther's Stolen Treasures

"Shopping" in other people's rooms for jewelry, clothing, pictures, or decorative pillows was a favorite activity for Esther. She would gather up her treasures and return to her room where she would deposit them in her drawers, under her bed or sofa, or under her pillows, and Esther's room was the first place we would look for missing items.

It's difficult to know if Esther realized she was taking something that didn't belong to her, or if she felt she had found an item that she recognized as her own and was bringing it back to her room to hide it in order to prevent it from being taken away again. It really didn't matter what the reason was, we could not accuse her of "stealing," nor could we attempt to take the item away from her while she was present.

I recall one day she came hurrying out of Annie's room with Annie's new Christmas sweater clutched to her chest. Annie was loudly shrieking obscenities behind her, while trying to catch up with her to get her sweater back. I didn't stop Esther because I felt I already knew what the problem was and I knew Esther would tearfully swear that sweater was her own. She would also be quite distraught if I tried to take it away from her. Instead, I went to Annie and asked, *"Annie! What's wrong?"* I moved in her way to block her attempt to follow Esther and also to block her vision of Esther.

"IT'S MINE, IT'S MINE! SHE'S GOT IT! IT'S MINE!" she shouted as she pointed around me.

"Tell me what is yours, Annie, and I'll help you."

Annie angrily tugged at the sweater she was currently wearing because she couldn't form the words to tell me: *"My coat, it's mine"* she said and I could hear the anger was starting to dissipate a little as she searched for the words to tell me. The picture in her mind of what Esther took from her was already starting to fade.

"Oh, Annie, I'm so sorry you're upset about this. I'll get it back for you, okay?" I gave Annie a long hug and she relaxed in my embrace and began to pat my back as I was patting her back.

"Thank you, thank you."

"You sit down here, Annie, in your nice comfortable chair. Oh, I see you were looking at these pictures of your little dog. He is so cute! What's his name?"

I had heard this story many times from Annie, but I knew it would elicit good memories for her and help her completely forget the incident with her sweater. It worked again this time, and she happily told me about Boomer and how she loved him. I left her sitting comfortably, looking through her pictures and I headed to Esther's room.

I know that Esther doesn't actually spend much time in her room. She just used it for sleeping, and as a repository for her treasures, so I was hoping she was already out of her room by the time I arrived. She was still in her room, busy wrapping the sweater around a small pillow in her dresser drawer. I ignored what she was doing and gave her a big smile: *"Hi there, Esther!"*

"Hi, honey."

"Esther, I just wanted to remind you that we'll be having lunch pretty soon and I don't want you to miss it."

"I know, honey. Thank you."

I left the room knowing exactly where I would return to look for the sweater while Esther was eating her lunch. Since Annie had already forgotten about the incident, I would simply place the sweater back in a drawer for her.

We had a room in the facility that we had designed to look like a little store. It had a hat rack with several ladies' and men's hats on it, a dresser with lovely pieces of fabric, beautiful scarves, a table with baskets of necklaces and clip earrings, and a mirror mounted on the wall slightly lower than normal so some of the shorter ladies could see themselves in it. The residents could walk into the room at any time and take any of the items they wished. Esther would often cart off as much as she could carry to hide in her room, and we would then wait until she was occupied elsewhere to "restock" the store with the items from her room. This kept Esther happy and busy, and it always delighted the other residents to find the store and be able to take any of the items they wished. Remember what fun you had as a child playing "dress up"? That's what it always reminded me of when I saw these ladies putting the lovely scarves and jewelry on and admiring themselves in the mirror. Staff would often accessorize a resident's outfit with these items to make them feel and look more beautiful. If you don't have a place in your facility such as this, you may want to consider adding one.

The Cake In The Clothing

We knew Louise was a "hoarder" and we would often need to check her room for food items because bits of food hidden in her drawers could cause illness as well as draw ants to her room. It certainly would not have been safe for Louise to eat the half of a chicken salad sandwich I found in her nightgown drawer one day.

One evening I was assisting Louise as she removed her clothing to prepare for bed. As I helped her remove her big, bulky sweater, an entire piece of chocolate cake fell out of her sleeve. Louise responded with a guilty little smile, *"Oh, my goodness! I wonder where that came from?"*

All I could think was, *"What a waste of a perfectly good piece of chocolate cake!"*

Hoarding items is quite common with people who have dementia and should largely be ignored, unless like Louise, they are hoarding food in their rooms.

In facilities, families should have the choice of allowing staff to routinely go through the resident's belongings to search for hidden food, or the family should take that task upon themselves in order to keep their loved one safe. Since theft is a concern in some facilities, the searches should be conducted by two staff people, and of course, the residents should never be present or know that the searches have been done in order to preserve their dignity.

In their own homes, people with dementia can get just as ill from eating hoarded food as those elders in facilities, so their families must be alert to the practice of hoarding and take steps to ensure the safety of their loved one by having frequent covert "search and destroy" missions.

"Let Go! It's Mine!"

I came around a corner in the facility to find Bill and Don grappling over a cane and shouting at each other. They each had both of their hands on the cane and were tugging in an effort to get it away from the other. I felt that was a good thing since it was occupying their hands, and they were not hitting at each other. Each man clearly believed the cane belonged to him, and they were not going to easily be persuaded otherwise.

"Hey, guys. Let me help you get your cane."

I placed my hand on the cane and since they both believed it was their cane, and thought I was going to immediately give it to them, they both, somewhat reluctantly let go of it. I called on the walkie-talkie for an aide to assist me and then said to Bill: *"Let's see here, Bill. You know I can see how you thought this was your cane since it looks almost exactly like yours* (even though it looks nothing at all like his cane), *but I see Don's name on the side here."*

The aide arrived and I instructed him to assist Don and his cane to another area of the facility. Knowing both of these gentlemen had just finished lunch in the dining room, I was fairly certain Bill's cane would be found there.

"Bill, I think I know right where your cane is so come with me and we'll solve this little mystery."

Bill was still miffed about the entire event because he doesn't like to be wrong, but he follows along with me to the dining room. When I found his cane I tried to make it seem like it's a mistake anyone could easily make.

"Here it is. Boy, it looks just like Don's cane! You know, I think maybe you should paint yours bright pink, or maybe put some sparkles on it so nobody will ever forget it's YOUR cane!"

I was saying all of this with a smile, and Bill grudgingly gave a small smile, too.

"No, I don't like PINK! Maybe red or something."

"Yeah, how about red with racing stripes down the side?"

Bill's smile widened and the potential crisis was over. It was important that Don be removed from Bill's sight, because it would have been much more difficult for Bill to calm down with Don and the cane still in sight.

As I've mentioned previously, humor is a wonderful tool that should be used frequently with elders who have dementia as they often maintain their sense of humor for a long time, and it's a real "connection" with them when you can tap into it.

Eli's Praying Method

Eli was a physically fit gentleman in his 80s who had had a series of strokes which left him aphasic (unable to speak), as well as causing dementia in his brain. He was of the Mennonite faith and had lived on his family farm his entire life while raising his family of seven children. It had become necessary for Eli to move from the farm for various reasons, and he moved into the home of one of his unmarried daughters so she could help take care of him.

Gradually, Eli's behavior became increasingly erratic and many times he would become so frustrated at his inability to speak that he would lash out in anger and pound tables or the ground while struggling to shout one or two words which made no sense at all. Eli was also exhibiting paranoia with several family members and they had made the difficult decision to place him in the facility where I worked after he began getting lost in the cornfields which surrounded his home.

The family had not told Eli where they were going that day because they knew he would refuse to enter the car, so several family members accompanied him when they brought him to the facility. When they came into the building, we seated them for a meal and then one by one the family got up and left the facility, leaving Eli with us. They had surreptitiously brought along some of his belongings and placed them in his room, but when we showed Eli to his room, he became enraged. He went to the front door of the facility and stood in the corner beside it, making it clear he did not wish to be approached. We left him alone and went on about our business, taking care to always shield him from anyone entering or leaving through the locked doors. From time to time I would have a staff member simply walk up to him and offer a cup of coffee, hot chocolate, or some food which he continually refused with a loud, *"NO-NO-NO!"* We placed a chair nearby and simply made him aware that he could sit there if he became tired of standing, and after an hour or so, he did sit on the chair. After another hour or so he started to become restless, looking around the room from his chair and when one of the staff asked him if he needed to use the bathroom, he quickly said, *"YES!"* She escorted him to the bathroom, waited for him to emerge, and then escorted him back to his chair. Eli was appreciative of her help and rewarded her with a fleeting smile, so we then used this same staff person to later offer him another drink which he gratefully accepted.

After Eli had spent the entire afternoon on the chair simply watching everything going on around him (including a sing-along where everyone was having a great time), the staff person approached him near bedtime and asked him if he would like to lie down. Eli agreed so she then assisted him in preparing for bed. He spent an uneventful night and the next day one of his sons brought his favorite recliner to the facility and placed it in his room. He did not let his father know he was in the facility since he felt Eli would still be furious with him for leaving him there. When Eli saw his recliner in his room, he broke into a huge grin, went over to it, and immediately sat down. Then, as if he suddenly became aware of the meaning of that chair being in his room, he became sad and began to cry. We tried to make him understand that he would be there temporarily, "just until the doctors can get your medicine figured out," and he seemed to accept that and became more open and friendly to everyone around him.

Eli loved to tinker with and fix things, so we had our handyman bring him all sorts of small appliances or things that needed to be fixed. He never actually "fixed" anything but he loved to work on them. He was more than willing to be working almost all of his waking hours, as had been his lifelong habit, and nothing was beneath him. Peeling potatoes was a favorite calming activity for him. He happily assisted in crawling on the floor to wash scuff marks off of walls, shining windows, or setting tables, and he always enjoyed the hugs of thanks we gave him for his assistance. He began to settle into a routine in the facility and seemed to be content, however there were still some family members he would refuse to even look at when they visited.

After Eli had been with us for about a month, one of the evening staff mentioned that when she checked on Eli near bedtime, she found him sitting in his recliner reading his Bible as usual. But, for the past three evenings she had also noted he had placed a square piece of plastic on his head. On the fourth evening, Eli quite willingly went into the tubroom for a shower, and while he was showering, a different staff person emptied his pockets before putting his clothing in the dirty laundry. Not being aware of the significance of the plastic she found folded in his pocket, she assumed he had unwrapped a piece of food at lunch and simply put the plastic in his pocket so she threw it away. When Eli prepared to sit in his chair and read his Bible a short time later and couldn't find that piece of plastic, he became incensed. He couldn't make this staff person understand what it was he wanted, and the more he tried, the angrier he became until he was literally marching up and down the hallway, shouting and hitting the top of his head. The staff person called a co-worker into the hallway, and after seeing Eli repeatedly hit the top of his head, this co-worker recalled being told about the piece of plastic. They quickly searched through the trash, found the piece of plastic, and when they returned it to Eli he was immediately mollified.

I asked the family if covering the head was part of their prayer ritual but they said it was not and they were as mystified about it as we were.

What was important was that Eli felt he needed that piece of plastic on his head while he prayed, so it didn't matter if we understood it or not. It also spoke to the importance of staff communicating with each other about anything peculiar a person with dementia might be doing. We then notified all the staff of the importance of that piece of plastic for Eli, and it wasn't long after that when he simply stopped using it. More than just honoring the particular faith a person believes in and practices, it's also about honoring their spirit and what it is that is meaningful to them.

"Help Me! They're Going To Break In Here!"

When a person with dementia is fearful of something or someone, steps must be taken immediately by caregivers to alleviate those fears because the rational part of their brain is unable to step in to help them sort things out. This story about Nora demonstrates the lengths the staff were willing to go to in order to help her become calm again.

Nora was depressed when she came to our facility to live. She felt that she wasn't much use to anyone anymore, so it really didn't matter where she lived. Her caregiver could no longer manage her care adequately at home, and she was quite willing to live in our lovely facility. She would maneuver herself about the facility in her wheelchair minus the footpads by walking her feet forward, but she often preferred to simply stay in her room.

Nora usually had a negative view about the world around her and her caregiver reported that she had no living relatives and believed she had lived a rather sad life. Despite her persistent negativity, we attempted to include her in activities and engage her as often as she would allow in pleasant interactions with the staff or other residents in the facility.

Nora's room was quite lovely with a large window which looked out onto part of the lawn as well as some trees and a bird feeder. During the day when she elected to remain in her room during activities, she would sit in her comfortable recliner and watch the birds visit the feeder and would seem to enjoy her view. However, sometimes in the evenings it was a different story. Usually at dusk, Nora would begin to hallucinate about men hiding in the woods who she knew were going to break in and hurt her, and she would pull her call-bell frantically.

"I see them right out there! Do you see them? They're going to break in here, I know they will! I saw them, over there! It's three men!"

"No, Nora, I can't see anyone right now, but let's pull the blinds so they can't see in."

"NO! NO! YOU DON'T UNDERSTAND! If you do that, they'll just be able to get in here and I won't see them until they break in! They're coming to rape me!"

"Okay, Nora, here's what we're going to do. I'm going to take you to another part of the building, where they can't see you and there are a lot of people around to protect you. Then I'm going to immediately call the police to come out to search the woods. I promise we will keep you safe. Okay?"

"Yes! Yes! Please don't let them get in!"

We quickly learned to make sure Nora was occupied outside of her room in a group of people when dusk fell, and to have the blinds already pulled when she entered her room to prepare for bed. Even in the groups of people, she would sometimes look at one of the male residents and begin to accuse him of plotting to rape her, but keeping her away from the windows at dusk when shadows would trigger her hallucinations drastically cut down on the terror she experienced.

It was important that she take our promises of safety seriously or she would not be able to settle down, and the only way she would take us seriously is if we took her seriously. We were careful to never tell her she was imagining things or that it was just shadows in the bushes. She would usually be able to calm down and relax after she was surrounded with people and we reassured her that the police had responded and were searching the woods. When she expressed a wish to watch them searching from a window, we told her the police chief had instructed everyone to stay away from the windows until he gave the "all clear." She would visibly relax when that "all clear" message came from a staff person, and we could then engage her mind elsewhere before taking her back to her room for bed.

Nobody knows whether these terrors stemmed from an actual event in her past, or if they were the product of her damaged brain. Nora's caregiver reported she had been expressing a fear of rape for quite a long period of time, most likely since the start of her dementia. At this point in her life, it didn't matter if she was reliving actual events, or if she was imaging them, because the terror she experienced was very real to her and we needed to take steps to minimize the triggers and to allay her fears.

Delirium

Delirium (which has also been known as acute brain syndrome) is a condition that develops, usually suddenly, and is often due to an illness such as pneumonia or a urinary tract infection. The person could experience intermittent changes in many areas including emotional swings, increased confusion, disrupted motor movements such as increased falls, or they may suddenly become restless when they're usually sedate and vice versa. Any sudden change from that person's normal behavior or routine should be investigated as a possible sign of an acute illness. Sometimes the first indication will be a fall in a person who normally never falls, or you might notice drowsiness in a person who normally never naps. Sudden agitation or aggression could also appear when a person with dementia has delirium.

Since urinary tract infections are so common in elders with dementia, the first step is usually to take a temperature, although absence of a fever is not necessarily an indication there is no illness present. Collecting some urine to test for the presence of white and or red blood cells is often the next step. Observing the person to note any increased frequency of urination or signs of pain with urination is important information for the physician to have.

Aside from an acute illness, delirium can be caused by various other disorders such as oxygen deprivation, poisons, or imbalances in electrolytes or acid/base in the body. Delirium in people with dementia is usually always treatable and reversible when the underlying problem is corrected.

It's imperative to detect delirium as quickly as possible in a person with dementia because they can't tell you when something is wrong. The longer it goes untreated, the higher the chances for a serious injury such as a fall resulting in a broken hip or head injury. I recall when feisty, little Bea developed delirium when she was first admitted to our facility from her home. I believe it was only her third or fourth day with us. She was quite compliant with the aide when she assisted her out of bed that morning, but as the aide began to remove her urine soaked brief and pajama bottoms, Bea suddenly picked up a clothes hanger lying on the bed beside her, and began to beat the aide over the head with it, while accusing her of trying to rape her. We were able to calm and reassure Bea by taking her seriously and removing that aide from her sight to "fully investigate her." We then allowed Bea to tell us her story, and apologized to her for the actions of our employee. We needed to collect a urine sample to check for a urinary tract infection, so with Bea's permission and a careful explanation of every step we made, we obtained a specimen. She did have a urinary tract infection and once we started antibiotics, increased fluids, and gave her yogurt several times daily[1], she improved quickly.

Older women with dementia will often cause a urinary tract infection in themselves when they forget they should be wiping themselves from front to back after urinating. They begin wiping from back to front which spreads bacteria from the rectal area to the urethra, and since they are often not hydrating themselves adequately, the concentrated urine can quickly grow the bacteria and cause the urinary tract infection.

When caregivers notice any deviation from "normal" and take steps to rule out a delirium, they are helping to avoid a possible major crisis such as a fall with injuries or a trip to the emergency room.

---

[1] Given to reduce the chances of the antibiotics killing off all the "good" bacteria in the bowel, vagina, and other mucus membranes and causing a secondary infection. It should be eaten 2-3 times daily while the antibiotics are being taken. It must be yogurt with "live" or "active" cultures added.

"They Just Stole My Baby!"

There was another time when Bea's sudden agitation and aggression signaled a urinary tract infection. It was a Saturday morning when I received a call from the aide at the facility. She told me Bea had gone up to Janet after breakfast in the dining room, and had taken Janet's babydoll away from her and accused her of stealing her baby. Janet went everywhere with her babydoll and now Bea was claiming it as her own. This naturally resulted in a tug of war over the babydoll, and the staff intervened to remove Bea from the dining room by telling her that her baby was elsewhere in the facility. They brought another babydoll to Bea, but Bea said she didn't recognize that baby and she wanted her own baby back. NOW! She had punctuated her demands with kicks to the shins of the aide who was at least two feet taller and outweighed her by at least 100 pounds.

At the time of the phone call to me, the aide and Bea were sequestered in a small room with the aide standing in front of the door, and Bea frequently renewing her physical attacks in her efforts to get her baby back. I instructed the aide to tell Bea that the "official investigator" for the facility was on her way and would be there in just a few minutes. She was to reassure Bea that "the other woman" who had the baby was also being held there until I arrived. That explanation was successful in stopping Bea's physical assaults on the aide.

I arrived to find Bea sitting quietly in a chair but looking like a thundercloud ready to burst.

"Hello, Bea. I don't know if you recall or not, but I'm the official investigator for this building and I'm here now to get to the bottom of this very serious matter. Tell me what happened."

"Sonsabitches stole my baby! They just stole my baby!"

"Bea, have you talked to your sister in the past hour or so? I know for a fact she came in here early this morning to take your baby to the doctor for you. She was nice enough to do that because your doctor said it's not good for you to travel this soon after having the baby."

"She did?"

"Yes, she did. Now, I understand you were upset enough to hurt this person and I want your promise that you won't do that again."

"Well, wouldn't you, if they stole your baby?"

"You have a point there, Bea, but nonetheless, we can't have violence of any type around here, especially with babies around!"

Just prior to meeting with Bea, I had indicated to the med nurse that she should bring Bea's PRN[2] medication in to give to Bea. We needed Bea's calm cooperation in order to collect a urine sample as well as to avoid other outbursts. At the same time, I was prepared for Bea to refuse to take it in her agitated state.

The med nurse offered Bea the medication with a smile and said, *"Here you go, Bea. I have your medicine this morning."*

"I'm not taking that shit!"

I then gave Bea the reason I had prepared in case she refused. *"Bea, the doctor said you need to take this medicine every single day in order for you to get stronger so you can take care of that baby properly. Now, your sister will be back with your baby in a little while and I don't want to see you too weak and tired to take care of it!"*

"Oh, all right, I'll take the damned stuff."

She grudgingly took the medication offered and I crouched down in front of her, made eye contact, put my hand over her hand, and spoke to her in a caring,

---

[2] PRN or Pro re nata is a Latin phrase which literally means "for the thing born." It is commonly used in medicine to indicate "as needed" such as "You only need to take this medication on a PRN basis."

serious way. *"Bea, I'm so sorry this misunderstanding has happened, and I know how upset you must be. Can we go ahead and help you get dressed now so when your family comes back you'll be in fine shape to see them?"*

I needed Bea to agree to allow the aides to work with her to get the urine specimen and by validating her concerns, treating her with respect, and asking for her cooperation, she does agree. *"I guess so."*

I can see she's de-escalating from her anger, and I need her to be as calm as possible, so I introduce the idea of collecting the urine. *"Bea, today also happens to be the day when the doctor wants to do some more tests on you to see how well you're healing after having your baby. So while these ladies are helping you get all fixed up, I want you to go ahead and pee in a cup for me and we can get that taken care of today. Okay?"*

"Okay, I'll give you piss if that's what you want!"

She had that little grin back on her face and I gave her a hug before she left.

I tested the urine and found a large number of white blood cells indicating some type of infection. The physician on call prescribed an appropriate antibiotic that we were able to begin giving Bea that afternoon, and I instructed the staff to keep Janet and her babydoll as far away from Bea as possible all day. After an hour or so, Bea had forgotten the entire episode and we took great pains not to remind her.

A Nasty Surprise Attack

Anger and aggression are often a part of dementia, and caregivers must always be aware of their body language and choose their words and actions very carefully to avoid escalating any situation. This story about Guy tells about a time when the trigger for his aggression was never known but the nurse's reaction prevented more harm.

Guy had been a well-respected teacher his entire adult life, and he now required admission to our dementia-dedicated assisted-living facility. He was a sweet and compliant man who had a wife and three daughters who had a close, loving relationship with their father.

Guy had only been at our facility for a week or two when he suddenly displayed a new and disturbing behavior. Carrie, one of the nurses, was kneeling down on the floor in front of the stereo system attempting to find a certain radio station for the group of assembled residents. Guy, as usual, was calmly walking around the facility occasionally stopping to inspect an object or shake hands with someone he encountered. Carrie reported that with no warning whatsoever, Guy came up behind her, put his arm around her throat and violently threw her against the adjoining wall. Carrie was quite shaken but keeping her composure, quickly got up and stepped into the adjoining room which had a glass door so she could observe Guy, who by that time, was simply standing and looking at her. Carrie called for help on her walkie-talkie but instructed the staff to only enter the room and begin to quietly remove other residents and not to approach Guy. She opened the door and spoke quietly and calmly to Guy who answered her back quietly. He appeared just as he always had, with no sign of aggression whatsoever, so Carrie asked two other caregivers to bring him into an unoccupied room and engage him in a quiet activity while she tended to herself.

Carrie's reaction to Guy's violent action is what helped determine the outcome of that situation, and that's what will determine the outcome of every interaction with every person with dementia. People with dementia are always reacting to their environment, to some stimulus to their damaged brains, and we may never know what that stimulus might be. Almost always, they will give some warning or indication that they are upset about something, but in this case, we will never know what triggered this aggression in Guy.

The important thing to remember is that it's the reaction of the victim that will determine just how an encounter will end. If Carrie had displayed anger and stood to face Guy, it's probable that he would have continued in his attack. If she had run screaming from the room, he may have followed her to continue the attack. By remaining calm and doing something unexpected (not reacting to the violence), she stopped his attack by confusing his brain with an "abnormal" response.

When training assistants to work with this population I always tell them if they get into a situation where a resident has a tight hold on them and is hitting or beating at them, they should suddenly move *toward* the person rather than pulling away. This will confuse their brain as well as their sense of balance just long enough and they will be much more likely to let go.

I think it's safe to say that every caregiver working in facilities has experienced agitation and aggression from a person with dementia at some time in their working experience. It can be anything from a threatening raising of a fist and verbal warning to a sudden striking out. It's imperative they learn a safe and effective way of reacting to anger.

In a situation with spouses still living together at home, reacting to aggression or anger from their loved one's accusation with habitual verbal responses could result in a sudden escalation of the aggression with disasterous, possibly even fatal consequences. Let me give you an example of what I mean.

George and Martha have been married for many years, and over those many years they have developed a pattern of speaking to and interacting with each other in certain ways. Now George has dementia and is becoming increasingly "short-tempered" about every little thing that happens. Martha usually reacts by telling him something like: *"Stop getting so upset about it, it's just..."*

One day George cannot find his wallet and has become quite frustrated. He angrily accuses Martha of intentionally hiding it. Martha, who would never even *think* about doing something like this, who usually goes out of her way to help him *find* everything, responds to him with: *"Stop acting so crazy, you know I would never hide your stupid old wallet."*

Martha has just told her angry husband, whose damaged brain has led him to believe he's right, that he's "crazy" and then adds fuel to the flames by using the word "stupid." George becomes enraged, yells back at her that he's not stupid, and hits her. Because of his brain damage, George may not even be able to feel remorse for his actions. If Martha had been able to just stop and think for a few seconds before responding to George's accusation, that blow could probably have been avoided.

I'm reminded of what we were all taught to do before crossing the big, dangerous street as a child: stop, look, and listen. Martha would see that George is truly upset and angry, and that his anger is being directed at her. If Martha took a few seconds to "listen" to just how her immediate response might sound to this angry, unreasonable man, *before* she uttered the words, she would realize that his damaged brain would interpret it as a verbal attack upon him. She would then be able to change her intended response to something that would help calm and mollify him. Remembering her body language and tone of voice, she could say something like: *"Honey, I know you remember that I had your wallet yesterday* (even if she never touched it), *but I honestly don't recall what I did with it. I'll help you look for it right now. I apologize if I forgot to put it back where you could find it. Have you looked through the desk drawers yet? I'll go do that now."*

What Martha has done by taking the blame, even though she is totally blameless here, is she has started to defuse George's anger. By letting him think he may have a good reason for losing his wallet (and it's not that he's *forgotten* where it is), he can start to let go of some of his anger and focus on what she's saying and doing. Martha could begin to search for the wallet, chatting the entire time about other topics, and if George then forgets they are looking for the wallet, she has successfully redirected his thoughts onto safer subjects. Because of the damage in his brain, George *cannot* change, so Martha must.

With dementia, you truly can never predict what that person will or will not do based on what they would or would not have done before dementia affected their brain. It can become a game of Russian roulette, with the person with dementia assuming the role of the loaded gun in every instance where they become upset about something.

When aggression toward another person or escalating anger, almost to the point of aggression, has been displayed by a person with dementia, whether they are in a facility or at home, it must be considered a harbinger of things to come and that person with dementia should be admitted to a gero-psych unit for evaluation. The use of an appropriate medication can help to take the edge off that dangerous behavior. That's _not_ saying that every person with dementia who becomes upset and yells should be medicated. Changing your response to the incident and then redirecting that person into another activity or thought pattern will usually be enough to de-escalate the agitation. It's those times when the aggression is totally unexpected and unprovoked by apparent stimuli, such as in the story of Guy you just read, or those times when you feel fearful for your safety with this person, where you must take steps to keep yourself and those around you safe. Unfortunately, it's a sad fact that it's the men who most often receive the medications for behavior control since they are so much stronger than the women and could cause the most harm.

By learning to control your own words and reactions, you could prevent that simple annoying outburst from becoming that loaded gun, and many times you can avoid the need for medications to control anger and aggression. That being said, don't take chances by believing that increasingly hostile behavior can be manipulated away. If you see a pattern developing with this person displaying more and more frustration, anger or hostility, and you've done what you can to take the blame and redirect their attention, you must speak with the doctor about medications.

A Close Call

This is a story about an early time in my nursing career when I didn't know as much about how to interact properly with a person with dementia.

It was around midnight in the nursing home where I worked, when the night guard called to inform me he had found Patrick wandering in the common area that separated the assisted-living from the skilled care. Patrick had his coat and hat on and when asked where he was going he replied that he was *"going home--my wife is waiting for me."* Patrick didn't recall that he now lived in an assisted-living apartment and his wife had recently been transferred into the skilled care for her terminal condition. Patrick was already upset that the night guard had detained him while they waited for me to arrive. After I heard his reason for wanting to leave, I made the mistake of trying to re-orient Patrick: *"Oh, Patrick, your wife is just down the hall here in one of these rooms. Why don't you come with me and I'll take you to her room?"*

"No, she's at home where I left her and I'm going home now!"

I then compounded my mistake by trying to make him believe I'm right.

"Patrick, I'm telling you the truth. She's just down the hallway here, so come with me."

"SHE IS <u>NOT</u> HERE. I KNOW WHERE SHE IS AND SHE'S NOT HERE, NOW GET OUT OF MY WAY!"

"Patrick, I know you don't remember, but your wife IS in one of these rooms, and if you leave here, she won't know where you are. Come with me and I'll take you to her."

Patrick suddenly lunged toward me and grabbed me by my throat while saying through gritted teeth: *"I TOLD YOU SHE'S NOT HERE AND I'M NOT GOING WITH YOU!"*

Lucky for me, the guard was standing beside me and was bigger and stronger than Patrick, and another guard had just joined us. Together, the two of them managed to break his hold on my neck in just a few seconds. I wisely decided to leave the area since the guards had succeeded in calming Patrick and were talking quietly to him about walking down the hall. I felt instinctively that he would be calmer if he could not see me since I was the obvious focus for his anger.

Patrick finally agreed to walk down the hall with them, with no mention of the fact that his wife is nearby and they successfully steered him into her room. He remained calm the rest of the evening, dozing off and on in the chair at her bedside.

Patrick caused me no physical harm, but could have easily done so were it not for the presence of the guards, and I learned a valuable lesson in interacting with people with dementia. Unless a person with dementia requests to be re-oriented, it serves no purpose whatsoever to do so. It often only escalates their anxiety, fear, sadness, or anger.

I'm not sure what would have worked with Patrick that night, but possibly something like: *"Hello Patrick, how nice to see you looking so fit this evening. How can I help you?"*

He then may have said he was going home to his wife, and I might have replied: *"Oh, it's been so long since I've seen your wife. Tell me how is she these days?"*

Once he began to talk about her, he most likely would have relaxed enough for me to think up some excuse to get him to walk down the hall with me. I could have then taken him into her room without ever mentioning to him that she was a resident there.

I know that my inappropriate approach to Patrick, my inexperience and inability to correctly "read" his mood and ascertain his wants, resulted in his attack on me. Patrick could not be held accountable for his actions because his damaged brain was unable to find any other way to respond.

"I Want To Go Home NOW!"

"I don't want to wait. I want to leave NOW!"

EmmaJean was getting upset and none of my usual excuses or delay tactics were working. She was determined to leave the facility and go home.

"But EmmaJean, the bus won't be here for another thirty minutes!"

"I don't need a bus, I'll walk. I've done it plenty of times before!"

"Well, someone has to go with you and there isn't anyone available for ten minutes or so..."

"I don't need anyone with me, I'll go myself!"

"But EmmaJean, your sister is supposed to come today to see you and she won't know where you are if you're walking home!"

"To hell with her! I don't want to see her. I want to go home. NOW!"

I had run out of excuses and EmmaJean had run out of patience with me. It was time to change tactics.

"Okay, EmmaJean, let's go now! I'm going to just stop my work here and go with you because the rule

says somebody has to go with you. I'll do it now. It's a beautiful day for a walk anyway."

I made sure I had a walkie-talkie with me and I notified my staff by telling them: *"EmmaJean needs to go home <u>right</u> <u>now</u>, so I'm going to accompany her on her walk home."*

The staff knew that EmmaJean had lived her entire life in a small town about fifteen miles away. They were aware when I said that I'm accompanying her on her "walk home" that we would be outside the building. They also understand by my cryptic message that I would attempt to redirect her back into the facility, or someone would need to come and get us when she became tired from walking.

"Okay, EmmaJean, we're off on our grand adventure!"

I tucked my hand in her arm and we exited the secure facility into the beautiful summer day.

"EmmaJean, I don't remember which way to go, do you?"

"Yes, it's that way."

She pointed in the exact opposite direction she should really be traveling and that's important information for me to know in case she ever escaped from the facility. That would be the direction we should search first!

"Okay, EmmaJean, you set the pace and we'll walk as fast or as slow as you wish. How long do you think it will take?"

"Oh, not more than an hour or so. It depends how slow you are!"

She sets the pace at a brisk walk. I was glad to realize that we were heading toward a long gradual uphill, and I was fairly certain that she would be slowing down soon. I chatted with her about her home and her family, I really wanted her in a good mood when she ran out of steam so she would be more accepting of returning to the facility with me. I notified the facility which direction we were currently heading in such a way that EmmaJean wouldn't be able to understand what I was really doing.

"EmmaJean and I are really enjoying our walk, and we didn't even stop to take time to watch the ducks in the pond as we walked past! I'll check back with you in about ten minutes."

This was to tell them that if the walkie-talkie was out of range or couldn't get through, and they didn't hear from me in ten minutes, they should come looking for us in a car in the direction of the duck pond.

I could tell EmmaJean was already beginning to tire after about four blocks, and I had steered the conversation away from "home" onto other subjects she enjoyed talking about. We talked about how she spent summer days as a child on the farm, and she was in a much more relaxed and happy mood. She continued on for another two blocks and was by then walking at a very slow pace.

"Boy, is it ever getting warm out here! Do you know what I would like right now, EmmaJean? I would love a big old glass of ice-cold lemonade. Doesn't that sound good?"

"It sure does!"

"And what would you like to have with your lemonade?"

"Umm...I think I want a cookie."

"Boy, does that ever sound good."

She had stopped and was panting slightly from her exertions.

"I don't know about you, EmmaJean, but I'm getting tired from all this walking. Why don't we sit down here on this little wall for awhile and rest in the shade?"

We sat in the shade for awhile and then I saw an aide from the facility driving toward us in her car. She stopped and asked if we would like a ride, and since EmmaJean seemed to have forgotten her destination, I came up with a suggestion.

"EmmaJean, I'll just bet that we could go back and get some lemonade and one of those cookies right now. How about it? Are you thirsty?"

"Whew! I sure am!"

We returned to the facility and had our lemonade and cookies and EmmaJean was so tired from her long walk that she remained calm the entire evening. She even retained that calm during her usual sundowning time. All of the staff asked her if she had a good "walk" but they didn't mention "home." If EmmaJean had again decided she wanted to go home, I would then have suggested that her sister would be there soon, and she could ride home with her. That would have seemed like a good alternative to EmmaJean in her fatigued state, and then she would have eventually forgotten about it again.

"The Cows Need Milkin'!"

David had been a dairy farmer his entire adult life and he now resided in the facility where I worked. He was a quiet and gentle man who had a dry sense of humor but it often took a bit of convincing for him to show it.

After so many years of conditioning, David had a farmer's internal alarm clock that would go off at a certain time every afternoon. He would stop what he was doing and head to the nearest exit door to go home to milk the cows. The first time that happened, David had triggered the door alarm and was almost outside when the aide reached him. According to her story, she had told David he wasn't allowed to be outside and he needed to come back in. He stood his ground and insisted "the cows need milkin'!" When the aide wouldn't loosen her grip on his arm, he did what he thought he had a right to do. He hit her! In his mind, David knew he had cows to milk because he had just milked them that morning and he had better hurry home because any fool knows those cows couldn't wait. He had no idea why this person was attempting to keep him from his duties and since she wouldn't let him go, he did the only thing he felt he could do.

That aide learned a difficult lesson that day, and we learned to honor David's internal alarm clock because he certainly couldn't change it, nor did he see a reason to change. There would be no way we could convince him that he no longer had a farm, or cows to milk. In his mind, the cows needed milkin' and he was willing to go to battle for them. We would have to find a much better way to handle the situation.

So, from that day forward, we would assign one person to watch David near that time of day. When they would see that internal alarm clock go off, and he would stop whatever he was doing to head to the nearest exit door, they would intervene before he reached it and say, *"David! There you are! Your son just called, and he milked all the cows for you today, so you don't have to do it, and he said he'll be here to pick you up a little later!"*

"Well, now, isn't that nice of him?"

"It sure is! He's a good son. You must have raised him right."

"Well, I guess I did," he would say with a satisfied smile. Then he would turn around and return to whatever he had been doing before the alarm clock went off. It worked like a charm every single day.

By redirecting him in this manner, we maintained his dignity and he was calm and happy his cows were being taken care of by someone he trusted. And it was so terribly sad when David eventually stopped going to those exit doors, and he forgot about his cows needing milkin'.

It's important to remember that no matter what the behavior is that is driving you crazy today, it will eventually disappear, and you may actually find yourself wishing they were still able to do it.

It's Different When It's Your Own Father

It seems that all of the training and expertise I have in dealing with people with dementia simply vanishes when I'm interacting with my own father. I struggle very hard to keep the frustration and anger at bay when Dad says or does something to make life much more difficult for everyone around him because of his dementia. All of that baggage that we carry around with us from our childhood, from our very complex family interactions, keeps getting in the way of my being able to be impartial and nonjudgmental with Dad.

Several years ago, a physician told my mother that Dad had dementia. Based on his behaviors, from what I've observed, and from what my mother tells me, I believe my father has Lewy Body dementia. This type of dementia presents differently than Alzheimer's and you often don't see nearly as much of the short-term memory loss in the early stages of Lewy Body. Families will describe their loved one as being "in and out" with their cognitive abilities. They say that one day they're "with it" and don't even seem to have a dementia, and the next day, week, or hour, they can't recall how to use the telephone correctly. Dad often becomes angry at my mother for something she does or something he perceives she's doing, and he will remain angry at her for several days. He can usually recall his daily events when I speak with him on the phone, so I believe his short-term memory is still fairly intact. When he is having "a bad day" he does forget just about everything and becomes impatient and frustrated over it. He does have progressive memory loss and can get lost driving or walking in town, but if he were in the grocery store with my mother and became separated from her, he probably would not forget that he was looking for her and wouldn't leave the store until he found her. Then he would remember that he had gotten lost for some time and it would add to his depression over his declining abilities.

Depression is often seen in people with any type of dementia, and in my father's case, we are faced with the very real possibility of suicide. Throughout the years, Dad has lost several good friends to diseases such as cancer or heart disease, and his youngest brother died of Alzheimer's disease. He has always said that he would never live with a terminal condition such as those; he would just end it all by shooting himself. We have no reason to doubt that he would or could do that. He's a very tough man and as a child, I recall watching him pull his remaining five or six teeth out himself with a pair of pliers because he refused to pay the dentist to do it in preparation for dentures. None of the family doubts that he would have the guts to pull the trigger if he knew he had dementia, so we don't tell him. I know you're probably wondering why we just don't get rid of all the guns in the house. We feel we cannot because Dad has always been an avid hunter and fisherman, and at one point in his past, had even been a gun dealer. He still owns several guns, loads some of his own ammo, and is very capable of shooting a gun. Because he doesn't have the short-term memory loss, he knows where his guns are, and would become enraged if we made them disappear, and he would then simply find another method to put an end to his life.

Dad complains to me about his inability to recall things, and since I'm a dementia consultant, he has asked me on occasion if I think he has Alzheimer's. I truthfully tell him that he does not, and I offer up several other reasons why he forgets things. He's a non-insulin dependent diabetic and I tell him that if he doesn't keep his blood sugars under control, that can make him more confused. I also tell him that lack of sleep from his crazy dreams and a total lack of physical exercise will contribute to his depression and thus increase his confusion. He seems willing to believe these are the reasons for his forgetfulness. I don't hesitate to tell Dad therapeutic fibs in order to keep him safe because I know that telling him he has dementia would only serve to make him more despondent and would result in him taking his own life, and possibly harming my mother and sister in the process if he felt they too, were suffering.

The decision to tell the brutal truth is a very personal one that each family needs to make on their own according to their circumstances (but they need to remember that it will be brutal, it will cause much pain and suffering), and then in the case of Alzheimer's, that loved one will soon forget the bad news, only to suffer again if they are reminded over and over because their family feels they need to be re-oriented and continually hear the truth. As in Lynette's story in "Holiday Pins and Needles," telling her mother of her diagnosis turned out to be a good decision because it led to her mother being given the opportunity to make her wishes known. But, as her dementia progressed, reminding her over and over of that diagnosis would not be at all helpful because her damaged brain would then require being told what "Alzheimer's" meant, then having her experience the suffering of hearing the diagnosis over and over again.

While Dad doesn't have the very vivid visual or auditory hallucinations that can accompany Lewy Body dementia, he does experience lack of REM (rapid eye movement) sleep where he acts out his dreams and awakens more tired than when he went to bed. Thankfully, this doesn't happen every night, but he has been exhibiting this symptom for probably the past six to eight years, long before any other symptoms appeared.

Another symptom of Lewy Body dementia is an intermittent impairment of muscle control. It looks much like what people with Parkinson's Disease experience with muscle rigidity.

Dad was always very physically active, and a few years ago he began falling on occasion because "my feet just wouldn't do what I wanted them to do." Since my parents live on the west coast and I live on the east coast, I telephone them frequently between occasional visits, and one day when I called, the phone rang multiple times before Dad answered it in a breathless voice. He had been sitting on the sofa reading when the phone rang, and when he attempted to stand up and turn to walk, he said his feet and legs remained at the sofa while his upper body turned to the direction he wanted to walk, and he had fallen. He continues to fall on occasion, and has suffered multiple cuts and bruises, but thankfully no broken bones. Because of these different symptoms, the fluctuating cognition, the muscle rigidity that comes and goes, the very vivid visual hallucinations, and the absence of early, constant short-term memory loss, the families of a person in the early stages of Lewy Body dementia face a different set of challenges as caregivers of these elders than do the families of other types of dementia. I strongly urge every family living with any type of dementia to join a support group, and if there are no specific Lewy Body support groups nearby, attending an Alzheimer's support group can help in many ways. There is an excellent website support group for LBD at www.lbda.org if you have access to the internet.

Having a father with dementia has taught me many things, and I would like to tell you the story about my father because I believe it will illustrate many of the challenges a family faces with dementia, as well as help you remember that we're all human and we will make many painful mistakes. It was quite a rude awakening for me to find that my expertise on the subject of dementia was sometimes of little help to me as I became caught up in the emotions and turbulence surrounding my family.

Dad was the oldest of ten children, and he had to quit high school to help support the family after he told his father to leave the house and never return or he would kill him. He did that to help save his mother and siblings from the frequent beatings his father bestowed upon them. So my father became a surrogate father to his siblings at a time when he should have been finishing high school. When he married my mother, she also helped to raise the younger children in his family while my grandmother worked to support her large family.

My two older sisters were born, and after suffering through two miscarriages, my mother gave birth to me. I had severe jaundice and almost died from the Rh factor reaction, so I don't know if that's what contributed to my father's favoritism with me, or if it was something else. They went on to have two sons after me, but I held that "favorite" spot in my father's heart for many, many years--not such a wonderful place to be as a child with siblings who know the score.

Dad was a very strict disciplinarian, expecting orders to be obeyed without question and immediately, or suffer the consequences of a beating with a belt. Money was always tight and we lived in a series of rented houses in Minnesota until we moved to South Dakota when I was around nine years old.

I always admired the fact that Dad could fix anything. He once made a bicycle built for two for my sister and me out of bicycle parts. He painted it red and white, which were his favorite colors, and my grandmother made red skirts for my sister and me to wear with white blouses as we rode in the local parade. Another time Dad acquired an old school bus and outfitted it as a camper for the family to drive to one of the many lakes in Minnesota, so there were many good times as a family and as a child of this hard man.

In my memory, Dad was always physically, mentally, and emotionally as tough as nails. He worked hard in his business as a refrigeration, appliance, and small engine repairman, but never made much money at it partly because he was so generous with his many friends, and probably also because he had no role models for good financial decisions or saving for the future. His relationships with several of the siblings he helped to raise came to an end because he pretty much cut them from his life after they wronged him in some way.

The reason I'm telling you all of this is so you will have a better understanding of the man today who has dementia. As with every person with dementia, their life history drives their behaviors and reactions today.

Isn't that what drives many of our behaviors and reactions too?

I married and moved far away after high school, coming back to visit only every few years because we didn't have much money. I got to see a more tender side to Dad in his interactions with his grandchildren, and he has mellowed somewhat as the years have passed, but has always maintained that very stubborn and demanding streak.

Attending to Dad's various medical issues is extremely challenging because he hates most doctors, which goes back to when his first child, my sister Kathy, was born and developed an illness with high fevers which a doctor misdiagnosed and led to her suffering brain damage. Kathy continues to live with my parents and helps out with dishes and laundry, and is able to keep her room in order, but has vision and balance problems which, along with the brain damage, render her handicapped. Dad's opinion of every doctor he meets is based on that tragic event.

Dad developed prostate cancer a number of years ago and underwent surgery and hormone therapy which left him cancer-free but requiring an indwelling Foley catheter. He's very bitter about that and while he can still change the catheters on his own, he firmly believes he knows his body better than anyone else, so he suffers from repeated bladder infections because he refuses to see the warning signs or use any technique other than his own for managing the catheters.

When Dad started to display some periods of forgetfulness I would receive reports of them from my siblings and occasionally from my mother. I urged her to speak with his physician about doing some in-office testing for impairment, but we all agreed it had to be without Dad knowing what they were testing for because of the suicide threat. The doctor did do some tests, told my mother it was dementia and prescribed Aricept, which he continues to take daily.

About a year or so ago, my parents decided they wanted to move from Oregon back to South Dakota in order to be closer to my sister and to friends living there. My father insisted he wanted to use U-Haul trucks for the move rather than have "a bunch of strangers come in" and pack up and move his belongings. He had also asked that my sister find a place for them to live in South Dakota, which she did, and which he agreed to over the phone. He was familiar with the town, and the area this new place was located in, and even though it wasn't as close to my sister's ranch as he liked, he agreed they could move this double-wide trailer later if needed.

My husband Doug, my sister, and I all flew to Oregon to help with the final packing and the big drive east in mid-May. Despite her frail health, my mother had managed to pack up most of the house items. Her reason for pushing herself to do so was knowing that if she didn't get things into unlabeled boxes, Dad may decide there wouldn't be room for "unnecessary" items such as knickknacks, my sister's doll collection, or extra sets of dishes. Mom has spent their entire married life doing end-runs around his decrees, in order to have some things she desires, and this was no different. We had to "sneak" multiple concrete lawn ornaments onto the moving trucks because Dad had declared them unnecessary. For some of the larger items, he was told they belonged to Gwen, the sister in South Dakota, from when she had lived in Oregon for a short time, and would eventually be returned to her.

Dad and my brother Mike had both wanted to make the 18-hour drive straight through to South Dakota as they had both done numerous times in the past, but we stood up to them and declared we would be stopping at a motel for one overnight stay. Since there were four vehicles and my brother Mike was only driving one of them, they acquiesced. Dad had said he would help drive when Mike got tired, but we solved that problem by "forgetting" to include him when we went to pick up the U-Haul trucks, and since he wasn't there, he couldn't show his driver's license, thus he was not an approved driver for the trucks.

Everything was ready for us to arrive in South Dakota at the new home, and friends and relatives were prepared to help us unload the trucks the day after we arrived. We got a later start leaving Oregon than we had planned, and with four women on the trip, bathroom breaks were more frequent than Dad liked. He refused to leave the truck to join us when we stopped to eat (said he wasn't hungry), so we just enjoyed our meals and brought him a milkshake and french fries every time we stopped to eat. He was always grateful for those and did eat them, so it was a good alternative.

At the beginning of the trip Dad rode in the truck with my brother Mike, but Mike's patience was wearing very thin with Dad's repeated stories and complaints. In order to give Mike a break I asked my husband, Doug, who was driving the other truck, if he minded if Dad rode with him for awhile and he agreed. Doug is a very calm and gentle person and had not heard Dad's stories multiple times like Mike had, so they got along just fine.

I've heard from many families that the constant repeating of life stories (called reminiscence) is one thing that drives them crazy, but it is one activity that is essential to helping keep the person with dementia calm and happy. So Dad happily told stories for hundreds of miles while Doug patiently listened and laughed in all the right places, which was not easy for him to do since most of the stories were of hunting and Doug does not hunt.

We drove for about ten hours that first day before we finally found a town with hotel vacancies and we dropped into bed exhausted around 2:00 a.m. At first Dad refused to leave the truck, saying he would sleep in the cab, but we convinced him to go to the hotel room with Mom and my sisters. Once there, he refused to take his dirty clothes off and was going to sleep on the floor, but finally agreed to sleep on the bed, fully clothed, on top of the covers. He was awake and rousting everyone in the room by 6:00 a.m., then left the room to go find our rooms. My sister became upset thinking he would get lost in this unfamiliar place, but my mother said to her, *"Let him go! Yes, he'll probably get lost but he'll stick around the hotel and at least he's not in here yelling at us to hurry up!"*

I think Dad must have terrorized the desk clerk into telling him where our room was because he was banging on the door at 6:30 a.m., then fussing and fuming while we all threw some breakfast down our throats before leaving.

We arrived at the new place in South Dakota around 10:00 p.m. after driving the entire day and evening, and we were all exhausted. Dad took a quick look around, pronounced it was "nice," and we unloaded a few mattresses and bags of bedding that had been loaded onto the trucks last in order to finally collapse for a few hours of sleep.

I awoke the next morning to a beautiful South Dakota day with the sun shining and the birds singing. I was so happy we had finally made it and was looking forward to a full day of unloading the trucks and getting as many boxes unpacked as possible. As I walked into the kitchen, Dad was coming in from outside shaking his head and looking downright grim. *"Nope, I don't like it here. I'm not staying so we won't be unloading the trucks."*

He had walked around the very small trailer park located on a hill overlooking the town, and decided it was *"like living in a goddamn fishbowl."* He didn't see that the physical position of this double-wide was actually quite similar to the single-wide he had just left in Oregon (except that he had owned that piece of property, and it wasn't in a trailer park) but the proximity of other buildings was quite similar. My attempts at pointing out the beautiful view, the deer I saw just outside the window, the fact they were on the end, so nobody would be on the other side did nothing to help him see anything at all positive about this place. He had made up his mind he hated it and was not going to stay. My mother caught my eye and motioned for me to call my sister to come and talk to him while she stalled for time.

Dad had decided he was going to drive to a town which was little more than a small dusty spot in the road, but was only about fifteen minutes from my sister's ranch. He planned to knock on the door of a woman whose husband had just passed away a couple of weeks prior to this, and ask her if he could buy her place. This "town" he wished to live in had no gas station, no grocery store, no church (just a little collection of trailers and houses in the middle of the foothills) and my sister had mentioned that at some point this woman may be willing to sell. It's times like this where I wished he DID have short-term memory loss!

My sister made it into town in time to prevent him from driving away, but he was adamant he wasn't staying in this trailer and we wouldn't be unloading the trucks here. I mentioned that we needed to unload the trucks because we had to return them or pay more money and Dad's response to that was: *"That's not a problem. We'll just drive them out to the ranch, unload everything on the ground, and cover it all with tarps."*

When my sister mentioned that she didn't have room for the three of them to stay with her, Dad's response was: *"I don't give a shit if I have to sleep in a tent. I'm not staying in this goddamned place!"*

In my business as a dementia consultant, I have advised countless families on how to interact with their loved one with dementia in such a way that it doesn't escalate the situation. I discovered at that moment that all of the training I have had, all the knowledge just flies right out the window when it gets down to the nitty-gritty with your own loved one. Of course, being severely sleep deprived, physically and mentally exhausted from all the packing, and driving, plus walking on eggshells around Dad contributed to my meltdown, but when it comes down to it, I'm no different than the thousands of other daughters/wives/sisters who are dealing with dementia in the family every day--and all of my training doesn't insulate me from the crises, or allow me to be objective.

When I heard my father willing to condemn my handicapped sister, and my frail mother to living in a tent rather than this lovely home they were standing in, I forgot all about the dementia, and only remembered all the thousands of times in the past where Dad had made major decisions based solely on what he wanted and to hell with what anyone else thought. I then spoke to my father in a way I had never spoken to him before, and in a way I hope I never speak to anyone again. I literally shouted at him: *"It's always about you, isn't it, Dad? It's always about what you want and to hell with anyone else's comfort or wishes. Can you stop for just one minute and think about what kind of life you're condemning Mom and Kathy to?"*

This had little effect on him and he continued to say he was driving out to the widow's place to ask her about selling to him. I again shouted at him: *"There you go again! It's still all about you. You don't care that that poor woman has just lost her husband. All you care about is that you don't want to stay in this perfectly good home."*

This also had little effect on him except for him to tell me to *"Shut the hell up. It's not your decision."*

I felt like my sister and I were playing "good daughter/bad daughter" because she remained calm, crouched down in front of him as he sat, her hand on his leg and speaking in a calm and reasonable voice. She did all the right things. There was a part of me looking in at the situation and seeing the stubborn, sad, broken-down old man before me and comparing that with the proud, strong, and fearless father of my childhood; the father who would have knocked me into next week for daring to speak so disrespectfully to him. He may have wanted to do just that to me at that point, but lacked the physical ability to perform that act. I was furious with him, and I was angry with myself for losing control, and I was incredibly sad. It was at this point that I wisely decided I was being of no help whatsoever. I had vented my anger, so I walked outside to join the guys who had escaped when the fireworks began.

My sister and her husband convinced Dad that the three of them would drive out to the widow's property to look it over, and my sister's husband, who is a model of diplomacy, would approach the woman if he thought she would be receptive to it. So off they went, while my husband and I went for a long, long walk. The guilt feelings crashed in on me immediately and as people do in such times, I cast about in my mind for a better way to have handled the situation. I could not blame or feel angry at my mother for not stepping forward in this crisis to put her foot down and tell my father that she and Kathy would stay right there and if he wanted to move out, then he could go by himself. That card could only be played as a last resort because he would do just that, then quickly become despondent and see suicide as his only option.

The guilt I felt at the disrespect I had shown, the anger that had erupted from me, and the hurtful words I had spoken lay heavily on my heart as my husband and I walked and talked.

The trio returned a short time later and my sister's husband held a thumbs-up out the window as they drove past, which I took to mean we were allowed to unload the trucks. When I returned to the house, I gave Dad a hug and told him, *"Dad, I'm so sorry I lost my temper and yelled at you."*

He quickly hugged me back and remarked, *"That's okay, honey, you're just like me sometimes."*

He forgave me for that trespass against him, but it took much, much longer for me to forgive myself.

The widow was not ready to decide about selling her property, and my sister promised Dad that as soon as the current house settlement went through, they would place that home on the market and look for something more to his liking. This crisis was over for now.

Maybe Dad was right in that I am just like him sometimes. I often know what I want, and I can be very stubborn about getting what I believe I want or need. But I don't have his volatile personality, I don't have dementia, and I know that no amount of stubbornness or knowing what I want is going to make Dad's dementia go away. This is the long haul as he moves into the middle stages of his dementia.

There is a part of me that is so thankful that I live so far away that I cannot help to manage the daily problems with Dad. Those burdens fall onto the shoulders of the family living there with him. There is another part of me that wishes I could be there to help ease those burdens to my family because I can see how their health needs are overlooked and overshadowed by Dad's constantly changing needs and demands.

There are so many families out there who are experiencing similar situations. They too, feel guilt, helplessness, frustration, and sadness at being far away. I can certainly offer suggestions to my family, and I often do, but sometimes I feel as if they're not taken too seriously. After all, I'm just the little sister. We just do the best we can and help out in whatever ways we can.

My hope in telling you this sad story about my dad, is that you will see nobody is immune from the trauma of dementia. We will all perceive any given situation in a way that reflects the "stories" in our own minds, and we will act based upon those stories and experiences. Sometimes we do the wrong things, and sometimes we get it right.

Educate yourself about the dementia, learn the tricks that work best with your loved one, and then be sure to take care of yourself. My ability to cope effectively with Dad and his dementia was gone when I allowed myself to become exhausted. You simply _must_ give yourself some attention and love, or you will be physically and emotionally unable to give your family member anything but anger and resentment.

The love is there. The laughter can be there and everyone will benefit if you strive for more of it. The mayhem will always be just around the corner, so my parting advice to you is to focus on the many things you love about this person, and take every opportunity to find ways to laugh with them daily.

Index

R

redirecting · 32, 33, 124, 242, 253

S

safety · 22, 35, 77, 81, 84, 85, 88, 105, 106, 107, 111, 113, 115, 178, 188, 205, 216, 227, 242

socialization · 78

T

therapeutic fib · 63, 133, 134, 165, 257

W

wandering · 36, 78, 81, 111, 244

CPSIA information can be obtained at www.ICGtesting.com
Printed in the USA
BVOW03s1355150914

366579BV00001B/1/P